Upon Arrival
of
Illness

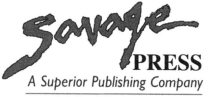
PRESS
A Superior Publishing Company

P.O. Box 115 • Superior, WI 54880
(218) 391-3070 • www.savpress.com

Upon Arrival
of
Illness

Coming to Terms with the Dark Companion

An Anthology of Hope

First Edition
First Printing

15 14 13 12 9 8 7 6 5 4 3 2

With thanks to John O'Donohue for inspiring the book's concept.

ISBN 13: 978-1-937706-04-3

Library of Congress Catalog Card Number: 2012916786

Published by:
Savage Press
P.O. Box 115
Superior, WI 54880
Phone: 218-391-3070
E-mail: mail@savpress.com
Website: www.savpress.com

Printed in the U.S.A.

TABLE OF CONTENTS

INTRODUCTION

Mary McGrath, being familiar with John O'Donohue's blessings, suggested the theme for this book. O'Donohue said he didn't like calling his poems, poems. He preferred the term, blessings. We here defer to him and trust that this is not so much a book as a blessing.

ACKNOWLEDGMENTS

This book would have been impossible without the help of Jessie Walsh, Marie McGauran, Amy Eliot, Mary McGrath, Laurie Hertzel, Karen Collins, Debbie Zime, Jaime Jost, Lynn Dufresne, John O'Donohue, and many, many others. Thank you all.

DEDICATION

For my niece Kelly

COVENANT

Katrina Smith

You ever think about rain? I spend a lot of time, lately, thinking about rain. It rains here and when it does the windows start to fog with moisture and I like to imagine that I'm looking at the world outside the way it really is. Insubstantial. Soggy with sentiment.

On Monday we had sun and I worked in the garden. I know what you're thinking. I don't love the dirt like you do. I know you're thinking I don't have the bone structure for wide-brimmed hats. I don't even know how to pronounce the word *dahlia*. Nevertheless, I bought this rose bush from a stand in the middle of the supermarket parking lot. It had two thick buds and a dozen leaves turning with brown, and to be honest I think the guy was glad to be rid of it. I carried it home with the eggs and milk and bread thinking, *I can find a place for this.* I spent the next three hours moving it around the back yard to get a feel for things and digging in the earth with a soup spoon I found in the kitchen drawer because I forgot about shovels.

Are you supposed to water plants after you plant them even if it's rained, or is going to rain? Can you drown something that way?

I don't want you to think I spend all my time on the subject of rain. There's a lot to do here. In the mornings before the sun rises I walk up and down the driveway and think about swimming in the lake. I read books. One day, I went into the shed down by the dock, where we kept our boat shoes and the lifejackets, which I have thrown away. The lifejackets, you'll be interested to know, aren't real flotation devices anymore. According to today's standards, we were not protected. Our childhood was nothing if not unsafe. It doesn't matter: there is a spider the size of a finger living in our old canoe, squatting between the ribs, pulling at a soft pearl the color of milk and exercising his own discretion. Having reclaimed what wasn't being used, I couldn't bring myself to ask him to move out. Who am I to say what belongs?

When it rains, though, I do look at rain, and at the world through the rain, until it stops. Sometimes I think maybe I am just holding my breath and if I let it out the mist will fall away and the water will stop and there you'll be, sitting on the lawn underneath the gray sky, eating bacon and eggs with runny yolks—like sunshine. Sometimes I wonder why, if I think this, I can't seem to exhale. Waiting to breathe out seems the most selfish indulgence.

Maybe I'm just after your bacon and eggs. When I do eat, I pull the crusts off of cheese sandwiches and dream of breakfasts.

Like sunshine and life jackets, I have given up old habits. I have done this for the sake of the future on recommendations I can only engage with. I imagine there are things inside of me that thrive on misinformation and if I am perfectly honest with myself, I am capable of sideways thinking. I wonder if I should kill this with love. I wonder if what is growing inside of me has perfect symmetry. I wonder if it will make holes like Swiss cheese until I am stretched membrane-thin and all that is left is yellow skin and a sense of quietness that I have always been unable to achieve in life.

I drove by a school on Thursday and outside there were four girls skipping rope, double dutch. Two of them were twins, wearing the kind of outfits twins do when they want everyone to know just how different they are. Doing what we used to do, showing the world that we weren't just doubled even if we looked like it. I parked my car and I watched them for a minute as they whipped the ropes around in the same way and chanted in the same voice. I didn't know kids still did that anymore, but it was as it always was: miss mary mack, mack, mack. All dressed in black.

Once, when we were five and you ruined my Rainbow Brite doll, I wanted you to die. This seems like the right time to make a confession, though I have no opinion on the subject of place.

I hadn't been here in a long time—never alone—and somehow, even though you are at home or at work or maybe in your own neighborhood grocery store, it seems like you are here, hiding in the back room, under the bed. You'll be jumping out from behind a door and sliding sideways behind the curtain when my back is turned. At the corner of my eye there is always the sensation of movement. I'm not quick enough to catch you. At my center, I am weighed down by pale stones. I do everything slowly.

I'm uncovering all kinds of old things out here. Out with the old, as they say. Except I took the lifejackets out of the trash before trash day. Stood at the end of the driveway at one A.M. in my shortest nightgown, digging them out of the bottom of the can. Past the rinds of my cheese sandwiches, which I did let the trash man take, thank you very much. I can let go of some things.

It is nearly July now, and July is always when we came here, kicking and screaming, ready to be bored with just each other. July is when we pushed shoulder to shoulder in the backseat of Don's station wagon waiting to get carsick. Do you remember? Promise to hold my hair back, you said, and I did. Forever, you said, and I said, Mom, she's bothering me, make her stop. But later I put my head down on your shoulder and I whispered of course, you ninny, I will hold your hair forever and you will hold mine too. I remembered this late last night and I thought, what would happen if you showed up here, because it is July and that is our migratory cycle, and I had no lifejackets?

I don't want to disappoint you. In the interest of full disclosure, you should know what I really did in the garden: I sat on a white gallon bucket in the middle of the weeds and I smoked cigarettes. I planted them burning end first all around my bare feet until only the very tops were left. I'll be checking back frequently. I'll let you know what they grow.

I think the rosebush is capable of saving itself. I left it by the front door. I'm hoping I'll see it shimmy down into the topsoil, right past the crabgrass. I expect it to burst out of that flimsy plastic pot any day now, brown leaves and all.

LYNNE JONELL

My heart breaks about eight times a day, on average. On bad days the number goes past fifteen.

I've taken to turning the phone ringer off when I go to bed, because heartbreak is worse at three in the morning. Defenses are low. And I'm not likely to get back to sleep after hearing, yet again, my mother's querulous, confused, increasingly desperate voice. Each time she calls she has a number of questions, but mostly she wants to know where my father is. I tell her he died seven months ago. I tell her he is in heaven. There is a pause as she registers this information.

"I *know* that," she says with immense dignity, "but why can't I reach him on the *phone?*"

Her illness is Alzheimer's, but I don't know when it arrived. Dementia is an uninvited guest, and a sneaky one. It creeps and hides in the pantry of the brain, nibbling away in secret corners. There are signs of its presence, but they are easy to miss at first.

Anyone can forget a name, for example. Someone under stress may cancel events for no apparent reason. And it's understandable that a woman who lived through the Great Depression would want to keep the refrigerator packed to bursting at all times, even if half the food is past its expiration date.

But the day I found the peanut butter in with the socks, I had a feeling we were in trouble.

How do you come to terms with an illness that destroys the brain of someone you love? You don't. Coming to terms is a phrase used in negotiation; it implies a certain give and take. But there is no give with dementia. It just takes.

It took Christmas this year. Two days after a warm and wonderful celebration with family, my mother had no memory of it at all.

Dementia snatched away the wedding of her granddaughter this past summer, with all its solemn Minnesota wonder and joy. It robbed her of the precious weight of her first great-grandchild in her arms. And the day she said goodbye to her beloved partner of sixty-six years has been permanently erased.

I will say this for dementia, though. It has improved our relationship.

When I was a child, my mother had many responsibilities and not enough time; it sometimes seemed to me as if she lived in a cloud of semi-permanent irritation. She bustled. When you were around her, things got *done*. For a dreamy child who was frequently distracted from the task at hand, it wasn't the best fit and I think we frustrated each other more often than others in the family.

When I was a teen, I was the rebellious child; there were heated arguments, hurtful accusations, wounded feelings that went deep. Over time, we developed a certain protective armor with each other. There was love and courtesy, but there was constraint as well, and many subjects were avoided by common consent. There was a certain caution, an underlying stiffness, as if the relationship had been starched.

The starch is all gone now. The protective veneer has been stripped away. Dementia takes and takes, but I am not sad that it has taken this.

There is nothing left but the love, now, and she is openhearted as I have never seen her.

She tells me "You were always a delight," and "I just remember the joy," and I know she means it. She can't tell me enough how proud she is of me, how blessed she is to have me in her life, how grateful she is for every little thing I do for her.

She doesn't remember the little things for very long, perhaps, but there's no question about how she feels in the moment. And I can keep the memories for both of us. For example, I'll never forget one day last fall, as I was about to leave the care center where my mother was recovering from a broken hip.

She was in pain, grieving the loss of my father, and afraid to be alone. She didn't want me to go, and my heart was wrenched, but I couldn't stay by her side forever. I had learned that it eased the pain of parting if I said a little prayer, so I bent over her wheelchair to do so.

And then she reached up to touch my head, and she began to pray for me.

She prayed with purity of heart; she prayed a mother's blessing. And as she prayed she stroked my head, my cheek, the back of my neck, with such sweetness, such tenderness, that I was almost overcome. I had the irresistible sense of being a child once more, held in my mother's arms, safe and warm and bathed in her golden love.

Suddenly I knew she had always loved me like this. I just hadn't always been aware of it.

Mother-child relationships are not always easy; there are some scars that are forever tender to the touch. But if there was any residual bitterness in my heart toward my mother, it was melted that day.

My mother has dementia; it is an illness I would not wish on anyone. And it is true that my heart breaks each time she calls. But there is something about a break in the heart that lets more love in; there is something about a crack in the intellect that lets more love shine through.

If this is the gift of dementia, I'll take it.

HEIRLOOM

Susan Thurston

As my mother awakened, she motioned for me to come to her side. The acrid scent of anesthetic drifted from her. With an elegant hand she drew me to her, and whispered, "Did they take it?"

I nodded.

"Come closer," she sighed. "I need to smell something beautiful."

I leaned down to her, and she inhaled the fragrance she'd given me a few months earlier for my 23rd birthday.

It was 1982, the Middle Ages of breast cancer treatment, when they rolled you into surgery, split open the suspicious behavior of your body, and if they found, with knife and lens, that those cells were doing what cells do, but without ceasing, they carved them out of you.

As mother and daughter, we rarely withheld anything from each other, and certainly not for long. We usually managed to tease out what needed to be discussed over coffee, or during an afternoon of shoe shopping, and always as we planted tomatoes or rolled creamy dough into sugar dreams.

That's how I knew she had been terrified—she didn't tell me about the tumor until the eve of her surgery. My mother was the most capable woman I knew, but she did not know how to handle this new valley in her life. If she could not deliver bad news on a platter, dressed with what could be done to make it right, she would not bring in her burden until the last possible moment.

She was not the first. My family's breast cancer legacy begins with my great-grandmother Susan. Susan's lustrous mane was a bodacious auburn during an age when all outrageous things were corseted, so she hid her embarrassment beneath a dusting cap. She nurtured capable daughters who worked hard, prospered, and celebrated even small triumphs by playing the piano by ear and singing in four-part harmony. She managed the binge-drinking husband—the horse knew the way home from the Corner Bar—and she made it clear to her daughters that a handsome face was not enough. Although a clear-spoken woman, when she felt the mass, she kept silent. When she could no longer keep silent because the pain twisted cries from her, it was too late.

Susan's daughter, my grandmother Elizabeth, was a bold woman, proud of the successful, boisterous family who gathered around her table on Sunday afternoons. My elders drank coffee with gusto from her heirloom china cups and dipped her homemade donuts in bowls of sweetened cinnamon. I listened to stories of how popped corn with sugar and milk constituted breakfast and supper during the Great Depression; how clothes would be picked open at the seam, turned and re-stitched for several more seasons of wear; or how some of their friends were never the same upon returning from "over there." My aunts and uncles would shake their heads, dazzled by their gains of good fortune. Then my grandmother would try to tell one of a handful of her oft-repeated jokes, but would be undone by her own laughter, its force so strong it would pull everyone forward, all of us cheering for her, urging her to cross the punch line herself. Breathless and hooting, she'd wave a hand and relinquish it to someone who knew it, while collapsing back into her chair, offering her dazzling smile.

When breast cancer came to her, she did not proclaim it; she mentioned it to her sons, allowed more glimpses of it to my aunts, and revealed it fully only to her daughter Mary—my mother. Grandmother wanted it removed and flung far from her presence. She did not want it to trap her as it had her own mother in a dry case of death. Grandmother survived the surgery, scoffed at feeble efforts of therapy, and died decades later on good terms with old age.

Within those preceding frames, after my mother's radical mastectomy, she agreed to experimental, oral follow-up chemical treatment that tagged her rounds of chemotherapy. She rolled a ball up and down the wall, again and again, to rebuild strength that never fully returned in her arm. She joked how she was grateful she started with a heavy head of hair, "So now I have just an ordinary amount." She presented commandments direct from the god named Oncologist who said, "Considering your family history, your daughter should get a base-line mammogram in her twenties." She insisted I do just that, asked if I were practicing my monthly self-exams, and sent me clippings about studies suggesting ways to minimize the risks of breast cancer.

My mother's cancer resided in the waiting room for nearly a decade; then, not long after my father's death, it came for another visit. She was content with a distant date offered for the surgery; I was not. After the biopsy, I stood at the nurses' station and said, "Find something sooner." The offending lymph nodes were removed within weeks. Episodes of cellulitis would regularly inflame her arm during the next dozen years, but cancer would not be the cause of her death.

More than 20 years after her first cancer, my mother traveled a modulated and gentle exit brought about by transient ischemic attacks. While sitting vigil, I opened the last drawer of mementos and tokens carried as touchstones throughout her long life: the picture of Dad too thin but beaming upon his return from Japan, Mother's Day notes scrawled in my brothers' little boy cursive, a picture of me on the day I was hooded for my master's degree. There were golden rings; a bone china coffee cup; pictures of us laughing on the front stoop of the farmhouse, our arms warm around each other's waists. I looked at a snapshot of my mother, lovely, taken within hours of the birth of my daughter Madeleine. In it, Mother bends over the hospital bassinet leaning close to her granddaughter, smiling, again inhaling something beautiful. I remember how she looked at me after the picture was taken and said, "A daughter's daughter is the most precious thing."

And then, there it was. Nested in a small box was the first prosthesis I thought she had tossed away long ago, hardened by her heat and action, its underside crusted by age. Its weight in my hand yanked me through the door of legacy. I looked at my mother, her breath shallow, her eyelids still. Taking her elegant hand, I leaned close.

Hours later, I walked out of the care facility; a full moon ached in the ink-dark sky. I stood in the nearly empty lot, watched the caretaker drive away with my mother's body, and sobbed.

During the years since my mother's death, flickers of cancer tease the periphery of my own body. I greet good news after each mammogram, and savor the words: Not yet. Not now.

My daughter and I talk about her maternal ancestors, their cancer journeys entwined in the sharing of their lives. I make donations. Sign pledges. Wear ribbons. I wish I could stand as a fourth-generation barrier between breast cancer and Madeleine. But I know all I can really do is take her hand, lean close, and breathe in something beautiful.

THE GIFT OF SHADOWS

Holly Harden

I once drew, with a black marker, an "X" on my left breast, just above the line of my bra. I drew the "X" for love of my mother's body, for the inch-long scar that wasn't there for much of her life, but has been since 2000, after the stitches and gauze and tape disappeared.

She had known for a long while that she had a lump. She didn't mention it until after. I was making a salad when she called late one afternoon. I didn't answer the phone; it was too hot in the kitchen. My eyes were burning and I didn't feel like talking. I didn't feel like anything, except maybe gorging myself on four-cheese ravioli or honey oat Cheerios and falling asleep on the couch.

She gave birth to three children, and breastfed only the youngest, a boy. Her joke is, since he was born, she can't ride a horse: it's too painful. But you don't like horses, is his reply. That's not the point, she says.

I have never seen my mother ride a horse. I have never seen her do anything where her feet leave the ground, except when she hangs wallpaper or gets into a car. She is not one to risk falling; her only fear is heights.

She left a brief message, which I retrieved after the salad and pasta were eaten and the dishes washed and dried. Her voice was tired and small. She didn't say why she called; she didn't sing her message to a patriotic tune. She said she'd call back.

I called her. I knew by then to ask, first, about her day and how she was feeling. She's reminded me often that I tend to focus on myself during our conversations. So I asked how things were going. She sighed, a vast sigh.

"I had surgery this morning," she said. She waited.

"I had a lump removed from my breast," she said.

"Which breast," I asked, like it fucking mattered.

"The left."

Ten years before she'd had a small lump removed from her right breast. At least now you match, I thought. I am pathetic.

"How big was the lump?" I asked.

"A large pea, maybe. But the incision is over an inch long."

"Where, in relation to the nipple, is the incision?"

"What does it matter?"

"It does, Mom. I need a visual," I said.

"It's above the line of my bra."

"Is it horizontal or vertical?" I asked.

"Why do you want to know? You're going to write about this. I don't want you to write about this." She was getting angry.

"Mom, just tell me."

"Neither. About a forty-five degree angle. And I am really pissed off. No more low-cut dresses. Nothing low-cut for the rest of my life."

"You're exaggerating."

"No, I'm not. They did not have to make the incision so long. This is a big deal. I don't think anybody gets it. I mean, I'm alone in this room, and I want to cry, and I have to put on this face because I work with these people. So after they cut me wide open and pull it out and put in the stitches, I went back to work. I thought, 'I know, I'll find Joan and talk to her.' Her office was locked. They told me she didn't even come in; her son drowned nine years ago today. I couldn't call her. How would I sound? 'Yeah, I got this little pea-sized benign thing taken out of my breast. My arm hurts. My breast hurts.' And in the meantime, she's thinking about her dead son."

"Mom, it's all relative. You can't compare pain."

"Oh, yeah? Well I can. Nobody thinks this is a big deal, but it is to me." There was fear in her voice.

"Mom, it is a big deal. Do you want me to drive down?" The drive to Rochester from Scandia is a little over an hour. No problem. I wanted to do something.

"No, no, no. Just paint your left breast black for a week. That would do it." She laughed, and then sighed.

"Are you going to tell the boys?" The boys are my brothers. I have two.

"Oh, I don't know," she said. "They won't understand. Men don't get it. I'd tell them and they wouldn't get it. What's the point?"

"Telling is the point. Telling is what matters. It doesn't matter how they respond. You need to tell them."

"I suppose you're right." Long pause. "Well, I should hang up. Greg just got home. He brought a bottle of wine and take-out. He's trying. I'll call you tomorrow night. We'll talk some more."

"All right." She hung up as I said, I love you. The phone beeped. I said it again, to anchor the words in the air.

The "X" on my left breast was neat and clean, unlike my mother's stitched skin. I used a permanent marker, a Sanford Sharpie Ultra Fine Point. It tickled. I drew it in my study, after I put the kids to bed, while listening to George Winston playing Howard Blake's "Walking in the Air," from *The Snowman*. In the movie, this is where the snowman, holding the little boy's hand, flies over fields and rivers and forests. When I've again heard this song, I've thought of the "X". The marker was not truly permanent; it did not remain, small and black, on my left breast.

I did not want to lose my mother to breast cancer, and I didn't. The lump was just that, and my mother is certainly alive. There was a lump before, and there have been lumps since. Those two were mine, excised a year apart, one per breast. I made my own joke to my doctor on visit number two. "Back to even 'em out," I said, and when she held up the shred of flesh which I'd asked to see, I promptly passed out. My lumps, both of them, were benign also. A blessing.

With the incision of that first scalpel, I stopped thinking I'd live forever, twenty years after I'd understood that neither would my mother. Breasts are life-giving, and to think of them as death-causing is its own particular darkness. The word "cancer" has been whispered, a now-present shadow in a lit life. Anything can happen. Anything might.

I like my breasts. Every day I run my hands over their contours, press down in concentric circles, feel for anything other than soft skin and firm tissue. And I talk with my mother often. I talk with my daughters, too. They are young women who dance with their shadows, draw "X's" along with "O's" on notes to boys, sing in the shower. They don't think about things like lumps, but they may one day. I hope to be there—if not next to them, then over the phone—should that particular shadow appear.

For now, the gift of shadows is their birth in light. If we are not alive, we won't die; because we are, we will.

THE BEING AND THE BREATH

Katie Maxim

There is someone in the farthest corner of my bedroom. I am unsure why he stays in the farthest corner. Maybe because he knows that the thought of when and if he will get closer incites more fear than if he actually was closer. I can feel the weight he carries. And I know he can feel the weight I carry because he is laughing and he only laughs for one reason. And so he feels, and he makes me feel, and this is how I know that he exists. He is intangible, inaudible, and in this lies his power. I am always alone with him. I am the only one who knows him. His name is not a single word that I can say out loud or tell someone or yell out angrily at him. I am unsure if he slipped into my home while I wasn't looking or if I let him in one day thinking I had power enough to make him leave when I wanted. I am unsure why he is in the farthest corner. I sleep with one eye open.

Tonight my legs do not work. I don't know why. I don't know which of these two things is worse. Sensing the presence of The Being in the corner, it is much like one of those dreams where you're being chased and your legs won't move, so I feel the instinctual desire to be able to run. But somehow knowing *why* my body isn't working properly seems almost more alluring than having it work tonight. Maybe if I knew *why*, I would be able to get back to that place I grew up in. That place called Health. But I am finding that Health is a mysterious place. Maybe it will be a long journey to get there. Maybe I cannot find Health without The Being. Maybe I cannot find Health by using my legs.

* * * * *

In Sickness, the dream of Health is linked to all other dreams. Some days the other dreams cease to exist and Health becomes the only dream. Some days there are no dreams at all.

On the days I allow myself to dream, Sickness becomes part of the journey back to Health. As I wrestle with him, I realize that the fibers of my soul flex and tear and build up again and slowly grow stronger. Many days drag on without any noticeable changes, but some days a thought or reaction that I don't recognize as my own comes springing forth from me, and I am struck with the evolution of my spirit.

I see the results most clearly after my encounters with the people Sickness has introduced me to. Some people I meet are wise. They speak of things they know. Not all of them know Sickness, but all of them know Love. They share their words with me, and it is like people sharing a meal, nourishing me. They are foods I know, but they are spiced and combined in new ways. I go home and repeat their words, tasting them, taking in their sweet aroma, and Hope gets healthier...even if I don't. Because of these people I grow.

Some people I meet are foolish and speak of things that they don't understand as they think they do. They speak when they should be silent. The words of the foolish cut at me and I go home and sort through them and bandage myself up and learn to hate the words and not the people who spoke them. I learn to remember that these people are frightened, in denial, hopeless...as I often am. Our humanity is the same. I pity them more than they pity me. Perhaps they have never known Love and therefore have none to give. Perhaps they have Beings in their bedrooms. Perhaps they have never eaten with the wise. Because of these people I grow.

* * * * *

Several years before I got sick, I started writing prayers on pieces of paper and putting them in a shoebox. Each New Year's Day, I read the prayers in the box. It is fascinating to see how many prayers get answered each year and how they typically get answered in ways I would have never imagined.

It is also interesting how quickly I forget I ever had a need after it has been met. If only the mind held onto the memories of all the answered prayers, Hope might thrive.

I started crying one day at the height of my illness while doing the dishes. I was crying for my body and my future and my family. It was a day I was not allowing myself to dream, and Sickness had become heavier than I could carry within me. It felt like Hope had finally stopped her labored breathing and widowed me. I closed my eyes and let my hands rest in the warm water as I cried. It was a small comfort. Too small to be of any help, but the only comfort I could feel.

As I stood there in my fear and my pain and my warm water, I felt something rise up and touch my hand. I close my fingers softly around it and lifted out a dripping scrap of yellow paper with a sentence still legible on it. I did not remember writing it and the moment felt long and peculiar as I looked down at my own handwriting birthed out of such an unlikely place as the dishwater.

"Remember that what you now have is what you once only dreamed of having." I re-read it as few times before remembering that I wrote the words years earlier after going through the shoebox and realizing some seemingly impossible prayer had been answered to remind myself that seemingly impossible prayers can get answered.

* * * * *

Hope is a living thing. It travels about, weaving through wise people's combinations of words, weaving around the soul as it tears and regenerates, and, evidently, sometimes, weaving up through the dishwater on a note you wrote to yourself in what seems like another lifetime when your body worked. Sometimes, Hope breathes easy and dances in all her color and glory, and sometimes she lies pale and lifeless beside you, her breathing so shallow that you find yourself listening anxiously for the sound of it. I don't know how the scrap of paper got in the water that day, but as soon as I drew it out, Hope and I both took in a long, deep breath, and we danced there in the kitchen.

* * * * *

I think that the reason The Being stays in the corner is because he cannot get any closer and still be who he is. Because even the slightest breath of Hope is enough to overpower him, and he knows it. As for the paper, I don't know what happened to it after I found it in the water fighting to float to the top, but I think it went missing again so that it can be found on another day when I need it most and in a place I least expect it.

WHAT'S NEXT?

Dorothy Sauber

Today it is easy to imagine I am not dying. In fact, I feel so positively alive that I wonder why someone somewhere told me I have stage IV lung cancer. This morning, I went on my routine power walk, pulled weeds, and made a list of tasks for the afternoon. Later today, I plan to meet friends for pasta and return home to read a few more of Emma Donoghue's short stories before calling it a day.

Perhaps I feel so positively alive because I am just that—still alive. On Sunday I learned that the last of the three friends of friends diagnosed with terminal lung cancer within days of my own diagnosis had died. Like me, none of these people ever smoked. Two of the three were women. Two of the three were younger than I am. The last to die was an avid cyclist and the forty-five-year-old father of two young children. Unlike me, all three had chemotherapy and/or surgery and radiation. But there is no comfort in any of our differences. The statistical odds for long-time survival, once metastatic adenocarcinoma is diagnosed, are sobering regardless of one's age, sex, or treatment choices.

Maybe I feel so alive today because I am already dead and exist in a newly attained state of afterlife. If dreams represent the real world, as some cultures believe, then about six weeks ago I made the journey out of this life and into another. I dreamed I was lying inside a crematorium. As I observed myself from the edge of the blaze, my physical presence dissolved, slowly turning into a pile of gray dust. Near the end of my dreamed burning time, when all that remained was the steel tray covered with molten ash and one white curved cranial bone, I suddenly realized I had surrendered myself for cremation one day early. In my dream, I recognized how true to my life my death was. In life I am forever ahead of time. It seemed only fitting that I arrive early to my own funeral as well.

While still dreaming, I had to decide what was next. Should I call a halt to the fire in order to enjoy one more day, even if all that remained of me was a pile of ash and one small head bone? Or should I accept my mistake and finish what I had started, concluding that losing one day wouldn't be all that significant? In the end, I let the fire burn on. After waking from the dream, I lay in bed for a long time absorbing how it felt to be dead, secure that all was as it should be.

At my fourth month cancer check-up, once again my blood work came back looking normal. My kidney function, blood pressure, liver, and pulse all suggested I had a good amount of health inside. "Are you really sure I have a terminal disease?" I asked my oncologist as I stood up to leave.

Without a pause he said, "That is the one thing we are certain of."

"How often do you think about dying?" a friend asked recently.

"Thoughts of dying are the bookends to my days," I replied. And it is true. Not once since diagnosis have I fallen asleep without remembering I am on death row, and I get plenty of reminders that I'm dying during the daytime as well.

Last week I ran out of check blanks and had to choose whether to order one, two, or four boxes of replacements. My newspaper subscription expires soon, and they want to know if I'll take the one-year or two-year deal. Early this spring, I admired the new varieties of Iris, but opted to plant snapdragons instead. Yesterday, I accidentally broke the stand off my alarm clock, and today I'm wondering whether to buy a new clock or go down into the basement in search of duct tape, a cursory implement of hope even in the best of times.

And there are plenty of larger questions about what's next. What is the best use of my time now that I know it is to be shorter rather than longer? Are there contributions I should be making to society or my local neighborhood? Does having terminal cancer mean I have a new mission or calling I didn't have before?

In the past, whenever I imagined my later years, I'd be spurred on in my fantasies by thinking of Mother Jones' union organizing in her fifties; May Sarton writing her most influential book, *Journal of Solitude*, in her sixties; and Lillian Carter, at age seventy, working with lepers at Godrej Colony in India. Writer Brenda Ueland trained for the Pikes Peak annual uphill trek in her eighties. My friend's mother-in-law, with two knee replacements, took herself to Paris at ninety-two, and then, because she was having so much fun, went on to Prague—all against her cardiologist son's advice. At age fifty-eight, I am surrounded by women who, after raising their children and finishing their careers, went on to reinvent themselves. But now my own wide-open prairie-of-a-future has been reduced to the size of a sandbox.

After my diagnosis, I finished the last two weeks in the school term before locking the door behind me. I had a good teaching career and loved my work, but as Charlie King sings, "Our jobs are not our work, and our work is not our lives." Being a mediocre college teacher, due to unpredictable missed days or compromised health, is the last way I want to spend my final days on this planet.

I am grateful that my college teaching career was not my life. In addition to teaching, I have parented, enjoyed plenty of travel and adventures, created art, and filled more than eighty, bound, black, journals with thoughts about books, art, and life in general. I also have a drawer full of file folders holding essays in various stages of completion about women authors, time spent in distant cultures, growing up in rural Minnesota, my father's death from Alzheimer's, and topics like beauty, human responsibility, and love. Last week I added a new file folder labeled *Cancer Essays* to the drawer.

Cancer Essays is not the book I was planning to write. But writing these essays is just the duct tape I need for my own questions about what's next. As I write these essays, I realize they are like travel writing. Thousands pass through Paris, but no two ever see the same city. Thousands write about dying, but once inside its city gates, no two walk the same path.

The time for imagining my magical crone years as a second Mother Teresa or another Virginia Woolf is over. But as long as I feel so positively alive, I can go on describing my own meandering through the streets of cancer sickness and the avenues of love and loss. I don't need to remind others that, regardless of whom we travel with, in the end we all travel alone.

SEAN JAMES MCGINTY

There was really nothing physically eye-catching or even memorable about the woman in the canopy bed. The bedroom, in fact, had more interesting features to it than the woman herself. There were huge French louvered windows across from the bed that let in the sounds and aroma of the crashing ocean below; the ceiling, cathedral in shape, was made entirely of long strands. At night when the room was hushed and still one could still recognize, just faintly, the pounding of hammers, the rhythmic resonance of saws, a man's voice shouting commands to his craftsman. This was no ordinary room, but a room where the impossible gave hope to those before Liana, old and young alike, who had come to pass on. Even in the dark Alanis could still make out the silhouette of a carved Madonna near the open windows. The woman gave her a sense of peace.

But at 45, well before the onset of the cancer, the mirror at her vanity had begun to tell Alanis about change, those tiny lines around her eyes which certainly the month before were not there. Nonetheless, narcissism had no place in her world these days. Alanis, ashen and pasty skinned with noticeable traces of missing hair, cocooned motionless beneath her new, crisp sheets. She had, for the last few nights, considerable difficulty falling asleep; then could remain that way for no more than twenty minutes.

For Alanis, it was all infuriating, to have the precision of her mind, always reasoned and disciplined, poisoned by the toxic effects of something as simple as *"lack of sleep!"* But now, undeniable signs the end was near: *an* isonomic; short-lived disorientation; the need for more and more morphine with lessoned reduction in her pain.

Closing her eyes, she forced herself to remember the good "... the blessings I've known in my life with the Twins, and Kiki," I have two beautiful daughters, identical twins, almost thirteen," her eyed welled with tears at the thought of not being there for the start of their womanhood. "And my husband Kiki that, through the years I have loved immeasurably, then loved him not for reasons unknown; then loved him again but differently and deeper than before." It was a pattern that had repeated itself all through their married life. Without warning, a physically powerful and intense shooting pain went through her entire body; so excruciatingly raw was the sensation she produced an ear shattering scream. "Kiki? Kiki? Please, I need your help! Now! Hurry! Please, I can't take it." Over the sounds of the ocean, there was no response to Alanis' desperate plea from downstairs. She was alone and excruciatingly hurting.

Quickly, the Demerol began to do its job. And Alanis' eyes shut tightly. Her breathing was deep with long, full breaths. Not the *Death-rattle,* as some refer to the *gargley* sound the lungs produce just before the last few breaths are taken. No, this was sleep for Alanis, and a deep one at that. Getting up out of her bed she walked quickly to the bay windows and drew in a deep breath. "Oh my God, that smells so sweet, she thought, and then proceeded to examine the skin on her hand, which was now smooth and free of spots and scabs she clearly recalled being there. She tried to remember when she had those spots and scabs, but, for the life of her she could not recall.

Alanis was surprised at the energy she had, and immediately set about planning all the tasks she wished to accomplish that day. Number one on the list was to purchase that blue suit and matching shoes in Paris she had seen in a magazine.

"It will feel wonderful to be back to my old self again." Paper, she needed paper because there were so many tasks to be done. On the way to the bureau, she caught sight of a young girl, no more than the age of the twins, in the mirror. The girl in the mirror was wearing the exact blue suit and shoes that Alanis had only seconds ago pictured in the window at the boutique in Paris. Shocked and stunned at what she saw, she could only stare hypnotically at the image before her. And then the girl in the mirror spoke.

"Isn't it lovely on me, Alanis?" queried the girl. Then Alanis saw, standing next to the elfish girl, her own image in the mirror: she was once again the pasty, thin as a bone cancer patient near death. "What... is... going... on ...here?" asked Alanis in a slow and deliberate manner; clearly terrified by what she was experiencing.

"Why it's the start of your change over, your transition, silly...." the mirror girl replied. In the blink of an eye and out of the blue, Alanis found herself on the other side of the mirror in the presence of the young girl. But the start was not a peasant one for Alanis: on her back, convulsing, gasping for air, bleeding from where she could not tell, a shriek, born from the pain of now being in the mirror and on the other side echoed, like a feral animal, throughout the land.

Kneeling next to Alanis, the girl reassured her: "It will be over in a minute, I promise." Gaining her deportment, Alanis sat up and saw it: the most incredible world she could ever, even in her wildest dreams image. The colors were fused, all in one incline, but each somehow retained its unique signature. Green was still green and blue was still blue. She felt in some sort of drug-induced state; something that left her feeling as happy as she had ever been.

She was not expecting to again find herself back in her bedroom. "I want to come back, please," pleaded Alanis "let me come back—I will do anything!" pleaded a sorrowful figure. "You will, but not just yet." A pained look, with knitted eyebrows, reflected the disappointment in Alanis. "Don't you get it yet, Alanis" asked the mirror woman." I am you, your Companion, to help you to come over. "To where? I don't understand. Over there?" asked a very bewildered Alanis. The woman in the mirror stood and was a clone, an exact replica of the sick Alanis.

"Okay. Let's see if you understand this: Imagine a fetus in its mother's womb: it can certainly hear noises from outside its self-righteous, interminable-like world this creature calls home. It can feel hot and cold, move, prick it with a needle and it feels

pain; overall, then, it can sensate just like you and me. Are you following me, Alanis?"

Quizzically, Alanis nods yes. "But, does it have any idea of the glorious place that exists, and awaits its arrival just four inches from it? Like you, it simply doesn't have the necessary tools to appreciate that world. Soon, it will. You will be just fine. You may not recognize me but I will be with you, your Companion. You, Alanis, are about to travel those four inches."

Opening her eyes, Kiki and the twins were hovering over her smiling with delight that Alanis was still with them. "God, how I missed you all," beamed Alanis. "Here, bend over and hug me, all of you. God, how I love you!" And with that, Alanis's Companion, oh so gently, took her by the hand, away from the hugs and love, and into the world of the mirror.

THE WHITE SPIDER

How I Decided To Have Both Breasts Cut Off

Mary Rehwald

Twelve years ago, when I was fifty-eight-years-old, a surgeon told me the white spider in my mammogram looked suspicious—that the biopsy he was scheduling would probably prove I had a malignant tumor in my left breast. He was right. Luckily, it was "Stage One" (small).

He recommended I have a lumpectomy to cut the tumor out, followed by several weeks of radiation, to keep it from coming back into the remaining breast tissue, and then 5 years of taking a drug called Tamoxifen. (I will call this 3-step procedure the "lumpectomy option" in this essay). Because he had cut out the tumor with "clean margins" (no cancer was found around the edges), he and I breathed a bit easier, and I decided I had some time to explore my options without panicking too much. Would I choose the lumpectomy option or schedule a mastectomy (removal of all breast tissue)?

I assigned myself a three-week deadline to do my research and make the decision.

During those three weeks, I read and underlined Susan Love's *Breast Book*, (it's still the best resource). I read other books. I went on the Internet. I interviewed an oncologist, a surgeon, a radiation oncologist, and a plastic surgeon. The oncologist ripped open his shirt to show me his blue dots from radiation he had had for lymphoma. He said to me, "you might not even have any cancer left in you now. One of your options is to do nothing more." The surgeon explained that she was certified to do what's called a sentinal node biopsy during whatever operation I chose, which would reduce the number of lymph nodes they would have to take out to see if the cancer had spread. The radiation oncologist drew me a picture of where the radiation beams would go—through my ribs and close to my heart. There could be side affects. The plastic surgeon did not know the cost of his reconstructive operation. I asked him to show me photographs from his work. He did. I knew from that visit that I was not at all interested in having reconstruction.

One of the most interesting things I read was the discussion at a recent American Medical Association Convention that had just voted to recommend the lumpectomy option over a mastectomy. One of the primary reasons seemed to be that breasts were so important to women. I didn't know if this was for making love or what.

In retrospect, I've decided the most important thing I did was to interview five women who had gone through the same agonizing decision. With their tops off. A nurse who worked for the doctor who did my biopsy asked women she knew in a support group if they would do this. They all said yes. I owe my final decision to their willingness to talk about their bodies and answer my questions candidly. I am deeply grateful to all these women who shared, in detail, what they went through.

People have asked me why I chose to have both breasts cut off when my lump was small and hadn't spread. Twelve years later I can easily remember ten reasons. First, if the cancer hadn't spread (which I found out later it hadn't), the mastectomy would be my one operation, and then I'd be done.

Second, there would be no or little breast tissue for the cancer to come back to.

Third, there would be no need for radiation treatments.

Fourth, taking Tamoxifen for five years could be eliminated.

Fifth, mastectomies lead to good survival rates.

Sixth, I had looked at the healed scars on three women's chests, and I had been comforted by how minimal they were, and how comfortable the women were with their decisions. I got used to thinking about that option as something that wasn't scary after I did that. I imagined my new body without my size D breasts—those big breasts that had gotten in the way when I played Beethoven's Pathetique on the piano. I imagined giving up wearing those uncomfortable bras that cut into my shoulders, whose straps kept slipping down my arms! Aah, a new body! Tubelike, yes, but still warm and happy.

Seventh, removing both breasts would be easier on my back which I had been having problems with since a bad fall years before. This happened.

Eighth, I had learned from my conversations and reading, that there is sex life after mastectomy. This is true.

Ninth, one bilateral mastectomy (removing both breasts) costs less than the lumpectomy option, and although I had insurance, I felt cost should be a consideration.

Tenth, I had been told the operation wasn't that painful, and this was true. Breast tissue is soft. It involves no bone. I got up from my bed after surgery and played a game in the waiting room with two of my friends.

So, what had seemed like an unimaginable option at the beginning of my research gradually changed into the most obvious one. I am well aware that most women make a different decision. In the U.S. at that time, 80% of cancer patients with my diagnosis were choosing the lumpectomy option but in the Duluth area it was 50%. I asked myself if that was because we were more pragmatic and down-to-earth.

One other wonderful thing happened during this time. My close friend Jill asked if she could come to my appointments and take notes and process the visits with me afterwards. "I want to learn about this, too, in case it ever happens to me," she said. Laughing with her and talking over how each doctor's visit had gone was the main energy that carried me along to making the best decision for me. This is something anyone can offer to do for a friend who is facing major decisions. I will always be so grateful to her for her follow-through and dependability. And her sense of humor.

Did I do the right thing? I know I did. I have certainly never regretted the decision. Before the call came about the spidery shadow, I had always wondered how I would respond to bad news knocking on the door of my passionate internal life.

I am so glad my no-nonsense community organizer self came to that door and took relish in getting into the fray. I am so glad my friends came forward to help me through those three intense weeks–they took my phone calls so I could research, they went to my doctor's appointments with me, they called and gave me much needed information and many contacts. They gave me confidence to do what was right for me.

PLEASE, DON'T TAKE MY SUNSHINE FROM ME

Jess Koski

I really like my prostate! I can say this with enthusiasm despite the fact that, five years ago, I only had a vague idea that I had one, and even less about what it did for me.

Irish poet John O'Donahue tells us that birth and death are very similar. "When you lie down to do it *(die)*, you will be able to do it with grace, a great serenity, and with a lovely courage, and a little excitement for where the new journey is actually going to take you."

That's all fine and good for O'Donahue who now knows for certain how true those words might be, as he died relatively young and suddenly in 2008 at 52, and though I'm slightly older than O'Donahue was, I am not ready to die just yet. I'm too busy watching and waiting, looking over my shoulder for that shadow to fold itself down in my direction.

There are several very different treatment options for suspected prostate cancer. They include radiation, surgical removal of the prostate, post-operative hormone treatments, and other, only slightly less nasty procedures. And then, especially if you are an older gentleman, there is "watchful waiting." As I was not an older gentleman at the time of my diagnosis, my doctor advised a more proactive approach—surgery. "You've got a lot of years ahead of you. Take care of this now."

The connotations here are ripe and metaphoric. When I remember to "watch" and to "wait," I can't help but wonder what it is I am watching and waiting *for*. Waiting for that spike in the PSA blood test that may signal more aggressive cancer? Feeling for some subtle pain in my clavicle or hip that certainly must be the insidious tendrils of cancer feeling its way through my body's ductwork? Watching the poker-faced countenance of the urologist as he completes a digital exam?

This urologist wants me to be vigilant. He wants me in for regular tests, biopsies, gentle scoldings. Mostly, he wants to take my prostate from me.

But I really like my prostate. "Sunshine" in the title of this essay is a euphemism of course. You, gentle reader, don't want to know about my erections. Of course you don't. So let's talk about it in terms of sunshine. The prostate, it turns out, is fairly necessary if you like erections (sunshine.) It's also useful if you dislike peeing your pants... as I do. Let's call that the "rainy day."

I enjoy conversations like this: "Look honey... It's another sunshiny day!"

But not like this: "Oh Sweetie... another rainy day? Well, throw those pants in the laundry."

In fact, I am a bit of a sun-worshiper; I like it to shine nearly every day.

So, I go on admiring the good work my prostate does. I eat a vegetarian diet, fairly free of dairy and chock full of garlic, onions, broccoli, spinach, and whole grains. I run marathons, and I meditate. I practice Qi Gong and send loving and healing messages to my prostate.

However, as the poet Andrew Marvell told his coy mistress (as he was trying to bring some 'sunshine' into her life,) "But at my back I always hear/ Time's wingèd chariot hurrying near." And I watch and wait.

It is fitting that sex and death are so finely intertwined here. I feel as though I am walking a fine line: Is it possible to have it both ways? Am I being selfish to want sunshine AND a long life? And is it self-centered to cling to my prostate even as I raise two young children? Should I risk gray, sunless days and rainy nights in order to potentially increase the odds that I will be there to watch them graduate high school, college, see them married?

Fear certainly plays into it. Most people who are diagnosed with cancer and offered the option of having it literally cut out of the body say, "Yes! Get it the HELL out of me Doc." Once a month, someone tells me about an acquaintance who's just died of prostate cancer. "Yup... he was doin' that watchful waitin' just like you and then all of a sudden it went into his bones and lungs and brain and POOF...gone... think about that."

My Arizona friend, Jim, had radiated "seeds" implanted in his prostate. Despite his area code, he sometimes struggles with a lack of sunshine in his life. After a few beers, over a campfire in canyon country, he will brood for long minutes and then exclaim, "Jess! Listen to me... don't do what I did. Don't listen to the doctors. You're better off dead."

And then, speaking of 'dead,' he continues, "A colleague of mine at the University just died. Watchful waiting..." his voice trailing off into the desert night.

So, I'll step up my vigilance for a while...carefully monitoring the color of my urine, and the subtle spasm deep in my lower gut as I lay awake, waiting, at 3:00 am.

And of course I'm different. I am not like that guy who died. He did something wrong, and I'm doing everything right. I think. I hope.

Marvell concludes his poetic argument with this advice:

> *Let us roll all our strength and all*
> *Our sweetness up into one ball,*
> *And tear our pleasures with rough strife*
> *Through the iron gates of life:*
> *Thus, though we cannot make our sun*
> *Stand still, yet we will make him run.*

And, just in case Marvell and I are dead wrong, and because I prefer the advice of poets over the calculations of the urologist, O' Donahue has the final word:

"At death...physical separation is broken. The soul is released from its particular and exclusive location in this body. The soul then comes in to a free and fluent universe of spiritual belonging. If you really live your life to the full, death will never have power over you."

EUGENIE DOYLE

Thirty women stand in a circle on a grassy shore of Burlington's Lake Champlain. It's July 2008, ninety degrees at 5:30 in the evening. Faces shine with sweat dampening hair of all colors, although, since this is a gathering of breast cancer survivors in various stages of recovery, not everyone has hair. They are members of Dragonheart Vermont, a competitive dragon boating team and tonight, they welcome "newbies," including me. The leader, with exquisite posture, a radiant smile and booming voice, starts, "I'm Linda, 18 year survivor." Everyone cheers. (We should. Linda organizes an annual dragon boating festival that has raised over a million dollars for cancer support services.) We go around the circle. I toss out my name and my measly one year which gets as loud a cheer as the two-time survivor who points to her left chest ("20 years") and to the right ("7 months.") She wears a red, not pink, scarf that matches her team jersey. Her arms look powerful, her face pale but glowing with a peacefulness I covet.

The coach, Linda's husband, gives instructions and we hit the water in two long, canoe-like boats for a session of rigorous drilling and racing. If someone tires, she pulls in her paddle. My seatmate totes a portable oxygen tank but is *not* the first to rest. There's joking but no whining. Self-pity? Absent! As she strides up the bank after practice, Linda points out a bench dedicated to a longtime member who recently died of BC. "Livona loved this view," Linda says, motioning to the setting sun, still water, the purple Adirondacks hovering in the distance.

Strength, acceptance, good humor in the face of loss and pain— that's about what you'd expect these days from a bunch of women cancer survivors. That, and a tremendous capacity to raise money to fight the disease. Breast cancer has emerged from the horrible, mutilating closet of the past and into a spotlight of hope thanks to women, their families and doctors who said, "Enough!"

Many Dragonhearters might describe their illness as not so much a "dark companion" as a flashlight showing a clear, though transcribed, path. They and members of other support groups keep the shadows of cancer at bay not with platitudes but with action and companionship that transform misery into the gentler conditions of compassion and peace.

But for me, this transformation has been tough. It's taken years and I'm not there yet. Cancer arrived as an invader, first with upsetting jolts: an unusual mammogram, then another, a suspicious white area in the mysterious sea of an ultrasound, the probing needle of a biopsy, the radiologist's look of concern, and finally, with the shocking diagnosis, *invasive ductile carcinoma.*

At first, I spent days getting to know "the enemy," reading into the night hoping for a clue to how and why and what now? I'm an organic farmer, a yoga-practicing believer in holistic health care. I hoped to avoid the strategy of surgery, radiation, drugs. But in Western medicine, cure requires conquest because cancer is painful, evil, ultimately deadly. No one counseled coexistence.

Before diagnosis, I thought I had been feeling fine, but after, I shook, lost appetite. Was the problem cancer or a sudden cloud of fear? I felt not denial, but doubt. Slowly, I began to think that if indeed there was a mutation held temporarily captive in my efficient catcher's glove of a breast, it might be a messenger instead of an enemy. My body was demanding attention. I lay in bed at night trying to decipher messages. This is what I heard: *don't be surprised. Breast cancer is common. Haven't you had yearly screening for this disease for years? Aren't you a woman and over 50, therefore possessing the two biggest risk factors? Why should you be immune? Aren't you stressed and exhausted by work and life?* I also heard this: *being afraid won't help.*

I felt something akin to relief. What I'd dreaded, what every woman dreads, had happened! I could stop worrying in the abstract and begin to deal.

I began to write and write, hoping to make sense of the treatment treadmill. At the hospital for surgery I felt I'd traveled to a cold, sterile country with no windows, in which the language is foreign but where everyone familiarly and frequently asks my birthday. My birthday! (One day, as I prepared for radiation, the therapist asked the rote question, when is your birthday and when I said, "today!" she asked again for the date and didn't even smile. Some of the cancer caretakers are showing battle fatigue.)

I saw surgeons, oncologists, nurses and technicians. I saw a physical therapist and acupuncturist for scar repair, for work on range of motion; a chiropractor for back pain. I even visited a hypnotist to help allay my fear of radiation (Didn't really work. I'll wager my farm that in 25 years this form of cancer-causing cancer treatment will be out-moded!) Most helpful were consultations with my beloved yoga/ayurveda teacher and with a counselor specializing in blending Western and Eastern views of health.

Yikes! This woman is nuts, you might say, and must have crazy good insurance! How could anyone eat up so much care? As treatment gobbled my time, I became fully aware of the resources I was using. I know that not all women in the world are so fortunate. I know women are dying all over the world from the disease. I know my "sisters" are dying down the road *in spite* of getting care identical to mine. We women are sensitive to things like this.

Instead of being crippled by "survivors guilt" women have emerged phoenix-like from this disease and its trappings in a flowering burst of compassion. We fully realize that we are mortal, we are the sick, the weak, the dying, even if cured of cancer! We know we want to live every day well and when it's our turn, we want to die well. We have seen our sisters, mothers, daughters mirrored in our own eyes. We have lost our hair, our breasts, our sexual identities yet have somehow emerged strong and desirable. Everyone seems fond of us pink-beribboned ladies and we love each other. Our sick bodies ironically have become the source of healing our spirits.

It has taken years for me to view cancer as a neutral result of imbalance in our lives, our environment, our genes. No more evil than the canary in the mine, cancer sounded a warning that I listen to my body and become compassionate towards others and myself.

So, is there a "dark companion?" Unfortunately, yes. Fear hovers nearby. Daily, I practice staring it down. Here's the kicker: Next week my husband starts treatment for prostate cancer. I will be his "enlightened companion," sharing with him my Dragonheart, yoga, and listening lessons: be aware, stay active, open your heart and treasure every day that we have.

WHITEWATER CANOEING THE RIVER CANCER

Caren B. Stelson

At 7:30 A.M., the phone rang. The doctor. I handed the receiver to my husband, Kim. His complexion turned from ruddy to gray. Then came the "c" word, "cancer," and our world turned upside down.

Cancer holds an icy grip on all of us. Knowing cancer comes in many forms, knowing many who have survived them, does not help when you hear the word *cancer* for the first time in your kitchen. That morning, my husband was diagnosed with colon cancer.

Still, the doctor was encouraging—we had caught it early. An appointment with a surgeon was set for Monday. The surgeon, the doctor had said, was "a cracker-jack, one of our best."

On Monday afternoon, Kim and I sat in the surgeon's office and watched as she pointed at photographs and coolly explained the lab results and options for treatment. She paused between sentences to look Kim straight in the eyes. My husband nodded. A professor of Mechanical Engineering, he was mentally analyzing the evidence, calculating risk. I could see his mind at work.

Anxiety clutched at mine. I gulped down the information and tried to wrap my tongue around questions, but my words sounded distant in my ears. The surgeon glanced at me, gave me a clipped answer, then turned back to Kim. "I have an opening this Friday." She pointed to her calendar. "Would that work?" Unflinching, Kim took out his day book and penciled her in.

The drive home was heavy with silence. Afterward, Kim went to work; I called in sick and spent the afternoon researching colon cancer. Colon cancer, unlike other cancers is predicable; it spreads linearly. Unchecked, it moves from the colon, to the lymph glands, to the liver. With early detection, colon cancer can be cured. Aside from the usual risks of infection, blood clots, and the effects of anesthesia from a major operation, colorectal surgery has its challenges. Lymph nodes, blood vessels and arteries are in tangled proximity, demanding surgical precision. What's more, the narrowness of the hips in a male body does not allow for much maneuvering. There are no guarantees. Elimination problems and sexual dysfunction can be end results. *No guarantees*—we had three days to rearrange our lives, postpone work obligations, and get our affairs in order.

The next day at work, I confided Kim's diagnosis to a friend. She peppered me with questions. "Who had we talked to? What had the surgeon said? Why were we moving so fast?" And the ace card: "Have you considered Mayo." She wrote down the name of a friend's husband, a doctor specializing in colorectal cancer. "Call Sam."

Of course that's the process. Ask questions. Seek a second opinion. Even a third. But my researcher husband— the one who asks questions for a living—wasn't following this stream.

That evening, I sat on the couch next to Kim. "We've asked more questions buying a new car than we have of this surgery. Don't you think we should get some more information?" I held up a card with Sam's name on it.

Kim shook his head.

"Why not?"

Kim looked straight at me and ticked off his answers. "I need to get this cancer out of me. I want the operation over with. I trust this surgeon. She knows what she's doing. Look, I've been giving this a lot of thought." Kim closed his eyes. "I'm going to jump in the river and follow the current."

In that moment, Kim had transformed from researcher to Taoist.

But I was angry. Didn't I have any say in this matter?

Wednesday afternoon, in the middle of a meeting, Sam the Surgeon returned my call. In shaky layman's terms I described Kim's condition and asked for advice. Without hesitation, Sam suggested we seek a rectal cancer specialist since the malignant polyp was so far down in the colon. He encouraged me to get *all* our questions answered. I didn't tell him who was asking all the questions.

That night, I related Sam's advice. Kim clasped his hands in his lap. All my questioning, he said, was pulling him off course. He needed quiet space to mentally, spiritually prepare himself for surgery on Friday. Please, Kim begged of me, just let go and be with him.

Thursday afternoon arrived. Following doctor's orders, Kim drank a gallon of "Go-Litely," a diuretic designed to "clean out" the intestinal track. Kim disappeared into the bathroom. I tied on my sneakers. I needed a walk, badly.

The March air was clammy, the sky overcast with shifting clouds. The weather reminded me of my life at this juncture, somewhere between the dread of winter and the promise of spring. Tomorrow we would find out how the rest of our lives would unfold. If Kim's cancer could be contained, we would likely resume our lives, and the sun would shine. If the cancer had spread, chemotherapy would surely follow, along with its debilitating side effects and lifelong worry. From there, it was easy to sink into winter's bleakness.

I thought about praying, but words eluded me. I needed something— a visual, a metaphor— that would help me somehow be in step with Kim. A picture of a river seeped into my mind. Memories floated back.

Twenty-six years ago, Kim and I had had our first serious date—white-water canoeing in Vermont during the spring run-off. Kim taught me to "read the river," paddle in tandem, watch for rocks, ride the rapids. At first, canoeing was rough going. We even capsized, but we hung on to the boat. Eventually, we found a rhythm, leaned in, and paddled our way down steam. At the end of the adventure, we had fallen in love.

Several days after that magical trip, I received a card in the mail—now framed on my desk. On the front, is a sketchy drawing of two people in a boat, with the words: "A relationship is a canoe trip on the Great Snake River of Life. It's lovely just paddling along, but when you approach white water, you either have to abandon the ship or work together."

Friday morning, we sat in the sterile hospital prep room, waiting. Kim alternated between gritty smiles and tears. I wrapped my arms around his neck. I was there for him, completely. One by one, the nurses came in and performed their pre-op tasks. I tied the strings on Kim's hospital gown as if they were strings on an old Mae West life jacket before Kim climbed up on a gurney. Just as the nurses rolled him away, I squeezed his hand.

The Tao Te Ching says, *those on the way of Tao, like water need to accept where they find themselves; and that may often be where water goes to the lowest place, and that is right...*

We were pushing off. It was time to paddle—Kim in the operating room, I in the waiting room. We would have to find our rhythm, go with the flow, and paddle down the River Cancer that spills into the Great Snake River of Life.

NO GOODBYES

Jacqueline M. Rennwald

I have always looked forward to autumn. Some say summer is their favorite. And why not? It's easy. But, I'll take autumn. Things go dormant or die; plants wither and prepare for the cold. Animals store up and take stock. Some burrow beneath or fly far away.

Mom died in autumn. September 28, 1976. Back then, everything was red, white, and blue. It was the Bicentennial and she got into the spirit. She sewed outfits for me and my sister's Barbies, crocheted ponchos for the three of us to wear, all red, white and blue. She made toll paintings of the Declaration of Independence, ceramics of the Liberty Bell and Abraham Lincoln. She died of cancer. I was seven.

My birthday is in autumn. September 12. Dad says Mom always felt bad I never had good birthday parties because she was either sick, recovering from treatment or surgery around my birthday. She first found the lump just before I was three, and then had a mastectomy of her right breast.

The surgery happened on a Monday. Mom and Dad were in a bowling league Thursday nights. One of the gals on the team didn't believe Mom had surgery since she was bowling that night. Mom asked, "Do you want to see the scar?" See, Mom was left-handed.

I only recall my seventh birthday from photos. Mom was in the hospital, though no one believed how sick she was. Any grownups who did were doing their best to pray it away or pretend it wasn't so. The party was at my Aunt Duffy's. There were two birthday cakes. One chocolate, the other was yellow with a doll in the center so her dress was the cake. She was beautiful. I didn't want to cut it and ruin her dress. Was she naked under there? Would my brothers and cousins laugh when the cake was cut away? I was embarrassed for her.

Photos show me talking that day with Mom on the phone. Opening presents and with the white phone and curly cord, I told her about each gift. I don't remember what I got or even talking to her. I'd give anything if I could. I wish someone could have whispered in my ear and tell me to listen, savor, and *memorize* every word, lilt, and smile in her voice because it was the last time I would hear her speak. How I would savor those words, and play the memory back in my head each day. No possession now could match it.

Fourteen days later she died, and so ended childhood. We had reaped whatever she could give us to sow and learn. All that was left was to store and preserve the memories we had. That autumn, part of me and my world died, burrowed deep inside, or flew far away.

Of course, there were no goodbyes. In those days, children were the unwashed and disease-carrying kind not allowed in hospitals. The last time I saw her I was waving as my school bus drove away. That day, she would have a checkup, be told she developed leukemia from previous treatments, and check into a hospital. To this day, I wonder if she ever asked for us, ever wanted to see us one last time, to say goodbye. Or was she, too, one of the ones who refused to see how sick she was, and was trying to pray it away or pretend it wasn't so?

Just recently, Dad and I were going through some of Mom's things; jewelry, papers, and stuff. Dad picked up a small piece of paper and gasped. I looked and he was already in tears.

My Dad was crying. Sobbing, with tears streaming down his cheeks, wiping them away with the front and back of his hands. Slowly, he held the paper out to me. It was a Memorial Card from Mom's funeral. The Virgin Mary was on the front and Mom's full name, date of birth, death, and a prayer were on the back. Then, at the bottom, in my small, childish and misspelled print, were the words, "Momy come back."

It was spring when I met my husband. After years of wandering and going through life without any drive or goal, I met someone who was completely driven and awake. From the day we met, my life began to mean something and have direction again. There was no more aimless wandering, wasting time, and drifting. I sensed a reason to wake up. I found a new path. Life began to move. It was Chuck who helped me focus and get on with life. Mom would have liked him. To this day, I believe she had a hand in us finding each other.

There are times it backs up on me and I miss her. Times I've held onto the Snoopy doll she won for me at a carnival and cried. My wedding was one of those times, as was pregnancy with my son. So many questions, so much we could have talked about. I dread Mother's Day.

Then one day in April, Henry was born. I was thirty-four, the exact age Mom was when she died. At a time when she was fighting for and lost her life, I was blessed with having a healthy, new one. It would seem spring should be my favorite time of year, as that is when my greatest blessings have happened. But it's fall that taught me to prepare, and show me what I can withstand. I can wear through dark days and know I'll be fine. Mom's death is like a shield. With it, I can weather obstacles or challenges. I've endured one of life's biggest hurts. Since I've lived through that, I'll live through anything. I've become a person with a positive outlook on life. Maybe, I'd have been that optimistic person all along, but I don't know. I believe God already took his pound of flesh from me, my mother and my childhood, and in return has blessed me with my wonderful husband and beautiful son.

Cancer doesn't strike once and leave. It stays and scars. It ripples through the lives of those left behind. Holidays, birthdays, anniversaries, it lurks and darkens. It steals into a room like a chill and no amount of layers can keep out its cold. My life is no more special or worse off than anyone else's because of Cancer. This is simply one small story of how it has touched mine. It's made me strong to the point of cockiness, yet sometimes brittle, and able to shatter at a word, memory or song. My son wishes he could have met her. He has her eyes. I wish he could have met her, too.

It is crisp and beautiful here in autumn, with brilliant blue skies one day and tumultuous gray and windy days the next. Life changes in autumn, as did mine. The hard road of winter is always ahead to test our mettle see what we've got. I like that. Spring is where the beauty is, but autumn Minnesota makes us put on layers, square the shoulders and face what's coming.

BIRD WATCHING WITH MY MOTHER

Teresa Boyle Falsani

July 11, 2002: Although I knew it enabled my mother to remain more feeble than she should be, I agreed to take her car-birding. At seventy-four, she's battled knee surgery and depression, exacerbated by an eye condition causing double vision and imbalance. We all feared she was having little strokes. But not only her poor health convinced me to drive her in motorized, air-conditioned comfort. Voracious Minnesota deer flies and mosquitoes swarmed in the driveway, bouncing off the car windows, crazed by our scent.

On a nearby dirt road, I stopped, killed the engine, and rolled down the windows a few inches. Over the drone of katydids, a hermit thrush riffed in the woods. From the roadside brush, a yellowthroat taunted, but wouldn't show herself. The heat had driven all the birds back into the shadows. Like an impatient child, my mother grasped the window and peered into the bushes, her arthritic fingers curled over the glass. She identified a veery by its call before the flies discovered the open window and attacked. We rolled up and moved out.

My Mother's Hands

My mother drank Knox gelatin, telling us
it made strong fingernails. She wore
rubber gloves to protect her hands,
lathered on lotion like salve.
My mother's strong hands carried
heavy binoculars into the woods, rolled strips
of wool to braid rugs, sewed fancy
Sunday dresses for her daughters,
tailored suits for herself.
Wearing flowered garden gloves,
she planted phlox and iris
more glorious than the sun.

Today, she forgets to water plants
and fill the bird feeder, shuffling
from room to room looking for herself in all the mirrors.
Her gnarled arthritic fingers
can't work buttons and zippers.
I fold her sewing machine down
in its cabinet, take her chilled hand
and help her lie down while I make supper.

Later, setting down my fork,
I say brightly, as I do every night

on this visit, "I cooked, you clean."
And every night, she answers,
"Oh fine. I'd rather do dishes than cook."
From the shallow drawer beside the sink,
she lifts her yellow rubber gloves
and wrestles them slowly
onto each knotted hand.

At a nearby wildlife refuge, we sprayed on mosquito dope and ventured down toward the
lake shore. In the bay, two tiny dots bobbed in the hot wind. Between them, a mother loon
surfaced and swam toward us. We stood still and silent, watching her prod her babes with a
sharp beak, swim ahead and pause patiently for them to catch up. When a bald eagle's shadow
passed overhead, the loon spread her wings and hustled her babies beneath. My mother tot-
tered closer to the shore, eager for a better look. I reached out to steady her, caught in the
push-pull of role reversal, especially when she shrugged me off, with a sharp rebuke that she
was just fine.

"She's laid right down for us . . ."

We were heading toward open sea,
the channel swathed in fog,
my mother rigid on the deck bench,
knees pressed together,
gloved hands clutching binoculars.
The captain's voice on the loudspeaker
cracked like lightening through the mist:
We're hoping for a smooth ride, folks.
Rough seas yesterday and riled, but today—
looks like she's laid right down for us . . .
"She's *lain*," my mother corrected him,
still sharp at seventy.

Six miles out, we anchored off
a tiny island, rocking on gentle swells,
rising and falling like shallow breaths.
All around us, dozens
of feisty, funny-beaked puffins
swam and squawked, trying
to distract us from their mates
nesting on Egg Rock. When the sun
burned off the last of the fog,
I hugged my mother,

thrilled to see my first puffin
colony clearly, at last.

Ten years later, when we finally put
my mother in the nursing home,
she lay right down for us,
but oh, she was rough the night before
and riled, forgetting we'd grown up,
slapping us like cheeky children
full of back talk,
taking me down
a peg or two, young lady,
you'll be sorry
some day, young lady,
just you wait.
So we never expected a smooth trip
the next morning, a calm car ride, windows
rolled up against the bitter cold,
or that she'd lie right down on the narrow bed,
fold her hands across her chest
shallow rising, gently falling
and smile.

It was my mother who taught me how to identify the call of the phoebe and the ovenbird; how to spot tiny warblers skittering through the pines on their way to Canada, how to pause and listen for the rustle of rufous-sided towhees foraging through underbrush. This day, binoculars slung about our necks like talismens, we resumed that partnership, despite the distance and occasional misunderstandings between us. After the loons disappeared around the point, I helped her climb stiffly into the front seat, surprised when she thanked me because this was her first close-up sighting of a mother loon with chicks.

Black Bird

At first, I thought the dog
had caught the little bird,
because she clung upside down
to the white pine stump,
chirping over and over, as if in pain.
But no, she righted herself
and began to drill, hungry.
Later, I find her in the bird book,
my first black-backed woodpecker.

Next to the picture, I note the day
and place, to annotate someday
in my meager Life List. When I call
to tell my mother, the master birder,
she says she's proud of me,
though through her window
in the dementia ward,
she can no longer identify
even a chickadee.

Tonight, I look up at a zero moon,
and marvel how
that small black bird
could bring back my mother—
her bright eyes restored
and full of passion, still
fastened on the sky.

On the way home, I pulled over in front of my neighbor's sheep farm. In the field by the barn, a fat llama grazed complacently, as if she were not our local celebrity, our poster child of rural exotica. I pointed her out gleefully. Look Mom—you can really see some neat wildlife here in northern Minnesota. As my mother raised her binoculars, the llama stepped aside, revealing a newborn calf, spindly-legged and wondrous. We smiled, watching them nuzzle. A mama llama and her baby in a bucolic summer field, plus, a mother loon and her chicks in the wild! Elusive songbirds and biting flies be damned. I rejoiced, because I had delivered.

Delivery

Hearing those words—my sister's—on the phone,
whose voice breaks between them, "Mom's gone," and then
"I was with her, she didn't die alone,"
I think, delivery at last— her end
long overdue once the bright stars burned out
in her brain and left us all in darkness,
this cruel albatross of grief slung about
our necks, her days pregnant with emptiness.

It was she first led me into the greening trees,
where learned human voices make no sense
amid the lilting thrush and chickadees,
a riffing wind that hints of recompense.
Today, I hear my mother joining in the song
and finally understand—she's been here all along.

MEETING LADY C

Mary Lu Perham

The first meeting with her was brief, but memorable. "You have lumps in your right breast," the doctor said. "I'll schedule a mammogram." I left the doctor's office, unable to think of anything else. What if I had IT? I was in my early forties, newly graduated into a career in education and human services. Life had hummed along nicely, and I had assumed that would continue. Now this.

It had always seemed to me that most people never lived for long once diagnosed with cancer. Over the years, several acquaintances had died within weeks or months of their exploratory surgery. My own family was an example. This dark companion had visited uncles and cousins on my father's side. A few years before his death from pneumonia, my father had been diagnosed with prostate cancer. Was I doomed to continue the trend?

Over the next few days, I tried to keep things in perspective. Not everyone dies of breast cancer, I reasoned. Two older women friends, both cancer survivors, had had mastectomies, and they were both alive and kicking. I wondered how it felt to not have breasts.

"It's hard," one of them told me. "I was always proud of my boobs. They were still nice even though I was no longer in my prime. The worst part is, my husband doesn't touch me any more."

She laughed, but I hurt for her. At least, I wouldn't have to pay that emotional price. I had no husband, no ongoing relationship. As far as I was concerned, my breasts were unremarkable. Maybe it wouldn't matter. But, what if I met someone later on, and it turned out to matter a great deal?

The mammogram results finally came in. "The lumps in your breasts are fibrous tissue," the doctor said. I was one of the lucky ones. The dark companion had moved on. I was Scrooge on Christmas morning, spared by fate and ready to reform, ready to celebrate this happy turn of events.

Life went on, but I now felt a need for urgency. I might not have all the time in the world. At the end of it, I wanted my epitaph to read "She made the most of her life." Through a variety of jobs, from teaching to job search counseling to coordinating a community education program and doing clerical work for a Finnish cultural publication, I expanded my interests. I began working on family history and genealogy, and learned to play the Celtic harp. I also bought a computer and learned to use it. In 1993, I made my first trip to Ireland to trace my roots.

In 1995, Lady C called again. "You have cervical cancer," the doctor said. "I recommend a complete hysterectomy."

"Can you do it right away?" I said. "I'm traveling to Ireland in nine weeks. I've already bought the plane ticket."

I was expecting a lecture about it being too soon after surgery to attempt a long trip. There was no lecture, just a call back with the surgery appointment. I felt no fear, no panic, even though this time it was the real deal. I had cancer. Perhaps it was because I was wrapped up in the excitement of my next visit to Ireland. Or, perhaps it was because I had worked hard at living. When reading or hearing about someone losing their life to illness or an accident, I had reminded myself of my own good fortune. Remaining focused on the present moment, I had crammed a lot of living into the years since Lady C's first visit.

A week later, the surgeon assured me he had removed all the suspect tissue. There was no need for chemotherapy or any other medication. Given this second reprieve, my visit to Ireland was extra special.

Since then, I've had other medical issues, other surgeries. Fortunately, there's been no sign of Lady C. Still, each time a new symptom comes along, I prepare myself. The pain in my joints would it turn out to be bone cancer, like that which took the life of my friend Mel? No. That turned out to be arthritis. What about my recurrent anemia, a condition that so far, has eluded a diagnosis? Will the doctor discover Lady C hiding somewhere?

I don't want to meet her again. Since her last visit, I've gained more wisdom. Life is far richer, more joyful, than I understood it to be when I was younger. I've learned how to use the talents I was given and want to keep on using them. After many years of single life, I'm enjoying a relationship with a man who brings out my best characteristics. I don't want to leave that behind.

I must admit, however, that Lady C's been a useful companion. Thanks to her, I appreciate my blessings. And, she forces me to make my daily experiences meaningful. If this dark companion is what I need to fully engage in each moment of life, then I accept the gift, with gratitude.

OPERATOR, INFORMATION

Beverly Jovanovich

Dedicated to my mom, Louise (Ehnes) Jones.

On my mantel sits a turquoise ceramic urn that holds half of my mother's ashes. My sister has the other half. My mother had a cancer tumor on her face that grew until the skin of her cheek could no longer contain it, thus creating a large open wound that grew rapidly. My sister changed her bandage daily, as mom stayed in her home and my sister moved in to take care of her. We knew there was no hope. Her doctor had made a wrong decision about the tumor and the cancer had progressed before they knew it was cancer. It would only be a matter of time.

Eleven twenty-four P.M. on August 4th was when the time came for mom, with my sister and I at her side. She no longer suffered from the pain, for which I am so thankful. But now, I feel pain. It is not the same kind of pain she felt. My pain is in missing her.

When my sister and I had mom's celebration of life service all planned out, (we made up her memory cards, chose the music, talked to my pastor, and went through all her old photographs to make the memory boards), it was a good feeling to know how it was all going to come together. As I drove home down highway ten, I was excited about all these plans and thought, I've got to call mom and tell her what we're doing for her service.

Then the cold shock hit me, it was for her.

And now in the evenings when it first becomes dark, I want to call her to see what she is doing or what she did during the day. But 786-8192 is disconnected. Then I feel empty. I realize that part of my life will never be again.

One evening, I went over to the Blaine City Hall for a concert by a group of women called TAKE 5. I was just starting to do things again, as I hadn't felt like doing this, what I enjoyed when I knew mom was suffering. I felt guilt. It felt good to get out. They were putting on a wonderful performance.

And then, they sang the song, *Operator*.

The words go:

Operator, information give me long distance.
Long distance, give me Heaven.
Operator information give me Jesus on the line.

My eyes filled with tears.

I have this record by the *Manhattan Transfer* and have played it over the years. It never really had a meaning to it. But, I liked it. I thought it was clever. I didn't know how this song will now always remind me of mom, as we spent so much time on the phone, but now, even long distance can't reach her.

SCARED TO DEATH ABOUT DYING
or
"I'm not really afraid of dying; I just don't want to be there when it happens"

—*Woody Allen*

Chuck Bransford

When you get that diagnosis, whatever it is you most fear, death becomes the elephant in the room. Suddenly: you slip 'beyond the pale', planted in an uncharted world, and expected to figure out how to live again. Oh don't worry, plenty of people will have all the answers for you: from the oncologist telling you about chemotherapy, radiation and surgery as if nothing could be simpler, to all the natural healers who tell you to just breathe right, take their supplements, follow an exhaustive vegan diet and settle on chi kung, yoga, energy healing, or just a good old fashioned shamanistic extraction of the evil cancer. Everyone wants to help. No one can.

One word changes the life landscape forever. As a medical student, I imagined myself getting every illness I read about except leukemia—that was just too awful to imagine. I had an extra job performing bone marrow biopsies on unfortunate leukemia victims and it just wasn't very pretty. In fact, it was horrible. We were told never to mention the "death" word to patients. Somehow, with all these people dying it seemed like it had to be someone's fault—my fault, their fault, the family's fault, the environment—too much algebra in high school or not enough. Someone had to be responsible—God? Even when sixty percent of my bone marrow was overtaken by leukemic cells I couldn't feel it. I couldn't tell the good guys from the bad. To this day, I have no idea when the illness started. How do I fight something I can't differentiate from myself?

So for me, I carried this black cloud of existential sorrow that surrounded my illness and gave it meaning that no platitudes from anyone could take away. My hairy cell leukemia treatment was quite simple: a 1 week continuous infusion of a drug called 2 CDA and then 6 weeks of waiting to see if my white blood count-or the cancer- would come back. Aside from the physical question, where might I find meaning in life again? The luxury of future time evaporates.

The rebuilding process takes one through childhood and adolescence all over again. You must begin again at the center of your being, comforted by a heart and soul that has generation upon generation of past experience to tap into. Initially, when you are very ill, you are a child again- emotionally, physically, and spiritually dependent on those around you. As you improve, if you are lucky, you become an adolescent. You can sense hypocrisy everywhere, including in yourself. Boring conversations are not tolerated. You call people out. The cancer diagnosis makes you a sudden tragic hero. Once you get beyond this adolescent phase, if you haven't burned all your bridges, things get interesting.

Whom should I tell? I really didn't want to tell anyone (including myself). How can I tell my daughters? They had the audacity to believe me when I finally told them I was going to be fine. One of the strange and wonderful effects accompanying my cancer was that the more people I told about by illness, the better I became. Other people became exquisitely sensitive, conversations were amazing, and all the rules concerning normal civil behavior went out the door. People stood closer, touched more, and eagerly revealed intimate information about themselves. I became expert at reading faces. I could tell a person's cancer history in an instant. If their mother or brother or aunt had died form cancer, it was in their face. If there was great suffering, it was there, palpable between us.

There is this glorious time when a mysterious alchemy of healing burns away your defenses, and you are happy about it. You are a new creation. It's as if you are the Starship Enterprise and you just can't get your protective force fields back into place. You've lost your filters and it leaves you open to experience the world directly, just like true artists do all the time. I spent my time immersed in every art possible. I loved opera, principally for the pure emotion. Tragedy was music to my heart in all forms—anything that brought forth tears. I was refilling my well. I felt acutely intuitive, almost clairvoyant at times.

So what are the components of this mysterious alchemy of healing that can occur when we face our 'dark companion' directly? For me it is: Breaking down the barriers of consciousness induced by fear, friendship, keeping an open heart and an open mind, exposure to nature in all her grandeur, acceptance of the unknown, the arts (actively participating in them), good symptom control, the gift of unstructured time (but not too much), having a purpose (no matter how small or trivial it may seem) being loved (and actually knowing it), plus being able to love, and most important, having a hero.

One of my life's guru's was Kay Lindahl. I first met Kay, who was 35, when I was a young consulting physician of 32. She presented to my clinic panicked and anxious beyond belief. Her identical twin sister (who was also her closest friend and college roommate) had just died from breast cancer. In her grief, Kay wanted both her breasts off and ovaries removed, but she also wanted children. She was scared to death of dying—who wouldn't be? I remember feeling so helpless and panicky myself in her presence. Luckily, I could refer her to a trusted oncologist. 10 years later Kay returned to see me. I didn't recognize her. She was so poised and comfortable in her own skin. Kay faced her fears directly, married and had a family, and after many years of study she was back serving as our new hospice/palliative care Chaplain. For 7 years she provided the gift of healing to countless souls suffering in our St Croix valley. She did develop breast cancer, and as her disease progressed she became better at her craft. She seemed to become the essence of healing. As her body diminished, her spirit grew, and connected to the world around her. Kay taught me to face fear head on. There is no other healing path.

When Kay was near death, she asked me to visit her at her home—a beautiful hobby farm with horses and a border collie who herself was a great healer. Kay lay in bed covered by a scrumptious hand made calico quilt. She had called me to thank me for our years of work together and to be sure that I knew she held no ill will towards me for not recommending she have her breasts removed so many years ago. My sudden burst of tears revealed how much I still carried this guilt, and how thankful I was to Kay for recognizing it at this time in her life. We spent a remarkable hour together remembering our past joys and sorrows until she gently slipped off to sleep. As I left the room, I looked back one more time and realized that there was a giant calico cat sleeping next to Kay with the exact same coloring as her quilt.

As you may have guessed by now, when I was finally able to come back to work after my cancer treatment, I followed Kay's example, and became a hospice/palliative care physician. Now, if I am attentive and open, not a day goes by when I don't experience a healed person, especially when they are dying. You die as you live.

WEARING PURPLE

Connie Lounsbury

He wasn't her usual doctor. He looked more like a patient than a renowned oncologist, his tired eyes peering deeply into Donna's pain. "I'm her sister," I said as he extended his hand first to Donna and then to me. The report of her last tests from him - a few questions from her - all with his face buried gravely in her voluminous file. "I'm sorry," he said as he shuffled out, shoulders stooped. No cancer-curative vials to take home this time. We did well, smiling blindly at the nurses as we left.

The big flat rock beckoned to us, warm and sunny, between the clinic door and my smoke-free car. We sat down. Fear gnawed holes in my soul as I sat there thinking about tomorrow's sorrow. Donna smoked one whole cigarette in silence, and then lit up another.

"He did say 'weeks,' didn't he?" she finally asked.

"They don't know for sure," I said. "You could have more time than that." I couldn't cry unless she did. That was her rule.

"My birthday is in ten weeks."

"I know." *Only 48.*

"I wanted at least another year."

"Me, too."

She lifted her chin and blew smoke into the beautiful Minnesota morning. "There's so much I want to do, yet."

"I know."

We sat there while she inhaled deeply, exhaled, inhaled again. She smoked slowly and deliberately, savoring—savoring that cigarette as if it was her very life.

Then she gazed into the distance and asked. "What kind of person am I?"

"Oh, Donna, don't you know?" I said. "Don't you know how special you are? Don't you know how much we all love you? You're a great mother, a loving wife, generous daughter and the best sister in the world. You're a wonderful person," I assured her.

Then it dawned on me. *She's finally allowing the question.* "Are you ready to meet your maker?" I asked softly.

Her tears came in great, gulping sobs, granting me permission to soothe my own hot, raw, throat. We cried and held each other—in public, in the middle of the day. Finally, she straightened up, blew her nose and said, "Well, I haven't been good all my life."

I explained that it doesn't matter; that God loves her and sent his son to die for her sins, so she could go to heaven. "I know all that," she said. "But what do I have to do *now* to make sure I'll go to heaven?"

Donna asked forgiveness for her sins and accepted the Lord into her life that day on the warm, sunny rock; then smoked another cigarette. On the way back to her apartment, I took the wrong turn somewhere, but Donna only laughed. We each had the Jenny Joseph *When I Get Old I Shall Wear Purple* poster on our walls, and had given ourselves permission to "act outrageously" now, since she was never going to get old.

She got worse. Hardly able to answer the door, she met me one day in a purple sweat suit, red hat and a brandy snifter in her gloved hand like the Jenny Joseph poster. She thought *I* needed a good laugh. And she never blamed me for not dying first because I'm older.

The New Year arrived. She could no longer stay at home. The dust collected on my shelves as she grew thinner every day when I went to see her in the nursing home after work. I couldn't help except to keep her company - and share my life - because she no longer had one, confined to the nursing home at 48, blessed only by her 98-year-old roommate's deafness. Her privacy was non-existent, her "things" crowded into half a closet and the top two drawers of a small bureau. All comforts of home were a lingering and yearning memory, seldom mentioned as I sat with her, talking, while my laundry piled higher at home and the sink filled with dirty cereal bowls from morning and another from evening when I returned home to cry again.

Today, her legs were more swollen. Today, she breathed with more difficulty as she sat at the smoking table, smoking one cigarette after another. What did it matter now? Her tumors grew in her huge white belly and her thin chest and arms looked like holocaust photos, and her head — angular, with teeth too large — and I loved her so much.

I pulled too-tight elastic out of her waistbands and offered to help her write last letters. She said she would do it herself, but I knew she wouldn't—because she couldn't.

She said she wanted to go home to sort through her belongings — give things to people who could use them. But she fell asleep during meals and her feet turned purple and she didn't mention her apartment again.

One day I said, "Donna, I love you so much. I will never forget you."

"You better not," she said. "or I'll wake you up during the night with the rattle of a stick against a rail fence."

My mail sat in stacks, unopened, in my apartment. I remembered to pay my rent. Donna urged me to tell her about my family, my job, my life as I filed and polished her fingernails. She saw the man sitting in the corner again—the man no one else could see.

They said Donna called out for me Sunday night but I had gone home to sleep and they didn't call me, and when I got there the next morning she could no longer speak. I'll never know what she wanted to say to me - or what she needed me to say to her. Her eyes just implored me silently - then returned to sweet escape of sleep while I read to her of God's unending love.

She died at 4:00 A.M. on Tuesday. In that quiet pre-dawn hour, the man that only she could see, must have stood and walked to her bedside saying, "Donna, it's time to go." I know she reached out with a radiant smile to our Dad, who went before her 15 years ago. I can see her rise from her wretched body and go hand in hand with him through the tunnel of light to Heaven.

The funeral is over. Everyone has gone home. I look in the mirror and see Donna's eyes in my face, and tears for her suffering and pain are now tears for my own loneliness. I know Donna is in a better place with no more pain, but I miss her.

The sound of a stick against a rail fence awoke me at 4:00 A.M. this morning and I knew it was Donna. It made me smile to know that I will see her again some day.

I also know that when it's my time to go, Donna will come to meet me, and because she always was just a little bit outrageous, I'm sure she will be wearing purple.

GREAT IMPACT

My Mother's Death by Illness

Shannon Esboldt

Death may be expected, but it is never predictable.

When mom first found she was sick again, we knew we didn't have much time, knew there were things to put into order. We knew there would be a degree of suffering and indescribable sadness. But never could we predict the impact that such a death—such a life—truly could render on those of us who survived her.

Mom and I weren't at peace with one another when her cancer re-emerged. As a mid-twenty something, I was experiencing tremendous inner-conflict and pain about my life and identity. I was angry at mom for both her contribution to it and her lack of ability to relieve me of it. For so many years and in so many ways, she had been a place of comfort and refuge. But the things I was facing at the time could not be caressed by momma's strong and gentle hand. She was a part of that with which I wrestled.

I was, I think, appropriately consumed by my "issues" and supposed that my struggle needed time, seasoned by counseling and prayer, to be worked out and settled before we would properly reconcile. The problem was that the time I supposed I needed was not afforded me. Just a day after New Years, following a painfully awkward Christmas together, I answered the phone to my mother's call with news.

"It's back...and it's in the liver."

Hardly can I say that I *received* the news. The moment it was spoken a shield of defense seemed to extract from an invisible place to shelter my being. I remember mom asking through the phone, acutely aware (and impressively respectful) of the distance between us, "do you want to come over?"

My very deepest regret today is that I did not run, RUN, to the house, fly through the door, and crumble in a miserable wreck at her feet, and in her arms. But I didn't have it within me then, which may have been a gift. For, with all that I had been encountering, it may have been the straw that flat-out killed the camel on spot.

Instead, I answered, "no" with the anticipated dose of shame, hung up the phone, and sat alone in a silent room.

What I began to think on in the quietness, in those infantile moments of the process of my mother's death, carried a realization that is hard to describe. It was the awakening that "ah, you too" are subject to the pain you've only *watched* other people experience. It was the beginning of the Great Impact that changed how I related to humanity.

When I began to share with people about mom's illness, no one seemed worthy of the news. It didn't seem like anyone could carry it with the weight it deserved. It took little reflection to conclude that the very best place, perhaps the only place, for my grief to be satisfied was with her—the one I was losing. Of course, that meant there was the painful and frightening pre-requisite of giving voice to my anger—to provide, by willingness of spirit, the opportunity to be heard. One wintery hospital night, an ironic scene unfolded, which answered the call.

I drove through downtown traffic with an uncomfortable mix of need and obligation frothing up inside of me. Mom was sick. She needed the comfort of family to meet her and to care for her. She deserved the honor. Yet I had been, and *was still*, so sick at heart, and she had not been able to meet me in my place of hurting the way I thought she should.

I took the elevator up to the oncology floor and felt my heart deeply pulsating.

When I arrived at her room, there was a quiet exchange of greeting. She was awake and seemed to have strength, but moving was painful for her. I sat in the only chair in the room which was at the foot of the bed. Dad must have left for dinner. It was she and I alone.

We argued.

In all fairness to myself (I'm still embarrassed sometimes about arguing in a hospital with a liver-cancer patient), she started it. She brought up the things we had between us...or, rather, the things that were the trigger of other things. I could feel the walls closing in around me as I desperately attempted to navigate my way through an impossible position. I was trying to give answers for years of unresolved conflict, things I hadn't begun to understand myself.

Ultimately, the best thing happened in that the bottom fell out. My composure failed me. My intellect capsized in the wash of my emotions. I gave up trying to provide words to explain and the proceeding moments are all I truly remember about that night. Placing my head in my hands, I moaned from deep recesses, "I'm just in so much pain!" And I sobbed terribly... on and on.

The room became still like a rain after the heat of day.

Quietly from her place in bed, momma begged permission, "may I hold you?"

I shuffled to her bedside. As momma sat further up and leaned forward to wrap herself around me, she gasped and winced. The effort was incredible. Within the minute, she murmured in my ear, "If you could feel how much this hurts, you'd know how much I love you and how much your pain matters to me. I *am* sorry." And I was sorry, too.

Under other circumstances I wouldn't have settled for our vague apologies. But I found there, and in the next steps that would usher us to her death, that my choice to forgive and to love were the most powerful choices I owned.

This is how I loved my momma.

I fixed-up the room she spent most of her time in, both cleaning and clearing and constructing whatever atmosphere of warmth could be attained. I came to the room often and visited with her and listened as she processed about end of life things.

When she became too tired to rise from bed, I would lay with her. Just lay and be near her. I'd drink her in and hold her hand.

When she became delirious and restless, dressed and undressed herself relentlessly, insisted on getting out of bed when she was too weak to support herself, when she kicked and fought and turned herself around and around on the mattress with confusion and discomfort, I sat beside her and I rubbed her back and told her over and over again how good she was doing.

When she came to settling, I covered her nakedness and stroked her bald head. I stayed and took my turn at feeding her eyedroppers of medicine to help keep her at ease.

I listened to her breath shallow and low until it was her last.

Not until her death did I recognize the pure and natural strength of the bond between mothers and daughters. Nor did I acknowledge the weight of a mother's sacrificial love. They are a part of the Great Impact. And I am never the same.

ON TRYING TO DEFINE ILLNESS

Amy Lindgren

Does illness ever really arrive? Or does it merely reveal itself, emerge from the shadows where it's stayed hidden while we've been going about our lives, never suspecting its presence? If that's the case, are we ever really free of illness? I've heard people describe health as the absence of illness, as if health had no defining virtue of its own. To be healthy is to be pain-free. To be without symptoms. With that definition, it's not a leap to say that to be healthy is to be unaware. Simply ignorant of the truth, of the illness that lies waiting for its cue.

My mother-in-law Alma was born in 1918 and survived the flu epidemic as an infant. She was so ill no one expected her to live; hundreds of thousands didn't. Since then she claims to have been so rarely sick precisely because she was so very sick then. She says she was inoculated from illness. Who's to say? It's a classic chicken-and-the-egg puzzle. Was she so strong that she fought off the flu even as a baby, in a kind of epidemiological foreshadowing of the Harry Potter plotline? If so, she received no mark of Zorro to prove it. Or was the flu so powerful that it changed *her*, creating an epidemiological super-human?

I don't know the answer, but I can tell you that she's one tough cookie, even now at 96. Still living alone and mostly making do in her cozy home on the edge of a lake, she can tell you stories that make your feet ache just listening. Everything she did in the 1930s seemed to involve walking miles and miles, hitchhiking when possible along the back roads of northwestern Minnesota. Perhaps the most amazing tale has to do with the burst appendix she survived while traveling home from her job as a maid at Itasca State Park. As she tells the story, she felt ill but needed to get home with her older sister Alice. The two walked and hitched and finally made the journey of several hours whereupon Alma collapsed in bed where she stayed for several days. And then she was back on her feet, back at work and onto the rest of her life. Until she had a hysterectomy in her 50s, that is. That's when her doctor asked, Did you ever have a burst appendix? When she answered No, he replied, I think you did. We found bits of it fused to things all over the place. They cleaned her up as best they could and Alma swears the operation cured a malingering sense of fatigue she had experienced since those days in the Depression.

Fact, fiction or fancy? You decide. I'm still working on my original question: Do our illnesses really arrive? Or simply emerge?

If we can't answer that, I'll settle for a different question: At what stage does an illness stop being an enemy combatant and start becoming a companion, dark or otherwise? And is it a grudging relationship or a wholehearted one? Can we ever really accept something that causes so much pain and wreaks such terrible havoc? Or is acceptance illusory? What point is there in accepting or not accepting something we can't control? It will happen in either case, so the point can only be one of ego. We want to feel control, so we control our own response. And that's supposed to bring peace.

Except I don't believe it does. It might bring truce, yes. But peace would be something deeper than simply a ceasing of hostilities. Peace has to be transformational, a new way of being altogether, not a return to the old way, before the illness announced itself. And not just a wary standoff with one side hoping to out-wait the other. How would that even be possible? I suppose that would happen when a person is healed of an illness, except I wonder: Would you ever trust your body again once you saw what it could do to you? You'd need more than physical recuperation to forget the original betrayal and move on with confidence.

But what about that other way of gaining peace, when one side overruns the other and the vanquished learns to live with the new rules? People with disabilities seem to have learned some of these tricks, although not always with equanimity. Take my father for example. He wasn't born with a disability but being hit by a bus at age 10 changed the balance. He became a gimpy kid with a leg that never really healed until finally, when he was 30, he opted for a voluntary amputation just below the knee. That was the year I was born, so I never knew him with two legs, but I did see all the coping it takes to operate with a prosthesis. He was the person who taught me to count my steps, literally, to make each process as efficient as possible. That wooden leg never really fit well and his steps were precious because of the pain they caused. So who vanquished whom in this scenario? Did my father declare victory over his body by throwing out the part that wouldn't work? Or did that leg, whatever landfill it ended up in, have the last laugh as my father limped painfully through life on its ill-fitting successor? Dark companion indeed. In his case, the companion was more like Loki or Kokopelli, the tricksters of Norse and Hopi mythologies. Mean, teasing companions always staying one step ahead with a new prank or joke to play.

The issue of companionship does raise a question. If illness might be the dark companion, and disability the prankster companion, what is perfect health? Besides theoretical, that is. Do we recognize health as a companion at all? Is it our bright companion, our friend, our reliable host? Or is it our ... nothing? The stepsister we keep in the attic and refuse to acknowledge because we don't need to? After all, if we have our health, what is there to talk about?

Feeling nothing doesn't feel like anything; we don't say we feel healthy unless we have something to compare it to. Have you ever noticed that a good workout is defined by the pain you feel the next day? We don't feel as if we're making progress in our bodies unless they hurt in some healing way. That must be why bruises are so irresistible to touch. You know it will hurt; you just want to know how much.

Maybe that's all we can ask when illness emerges, joins its steps with ours. We can't always bargain with it or make it leave. But we can push against it to confirm the one thing we really want to know: Does this hurt? Am I still here?

VIOLA LABOUNTY

December 3, 2011. She'd been sick for a while with pneumonia, they said. But it just wasn't going away. So they did an MRI to see what else might be going on. Then came the unexpected diagnosis, a tumor in her lung. Next began the waiting for more test results. Cancer, at the age of fifty-nine. It had spread to other areas. It was already in fourth stage. She had had no indication, symptoms may have been masked by her Lyme's disease the year before.

Now the oncologist was telling her it was terminal. It was too late for surgery.

She and her husband and son decided to go to Rochester, Minnesota, to the Mayo Clinic to see what her options might be. There was a promising one, a DNA treatment requiring a biopsy from her liver, (the cancer was there already). The risk of bleeding was less than 1%. She bled and was rushed to surgery to repair that, which went well. ICU for a few days, then a regular room at St. Mary's Hospital there. Her recovery was slow, so needed more testing, units of blood and potassium and pain medication for an old back surgery she had had years ago that flared up. She couldn't keep food down and her digestive tract wasn't regulating itself yet, so she was extremely uncomfortable.

Doctors kept saying, "Just a few more days." They were trying to keep her pain under control. Pain would come back as medication wore off and she had to tolerate it until time came for the next dose. She had continuous oxygen due to the remaining pneumonia in one lung. A procedure to remove fluid from around lungs, regular nebulizer treatments were tiring and caused her head to ache, for which she could have Tylenol. Her blood count showed there was more infection somewhere that couldn't be located. Meanwhile, two and a half weeks had passed and they were unable to treat the cancer with chemotherapy to keep it at bay. The Palliative care team said, "a few more days to keep pain under control first."

So, with that news, we headed to Rochester to bring support a to sister and brother-in-law who were terribly exhausted. Tender messages of caring encouragement were flowing in on the Caring Bridge site. But we felt we needed to be there with them. Involuntary tears escaped the corners of my eyes as we drove to be closer. We could only offer closeness and reassurance that they were in God's hands and under His merciful care. We still held onto the hope of this gene treatment two and a half weeks away to give her some quality time. People say it is encouraging, even at 4th stage.

After spending hours with her for two days of alertness and clarity, we had times of unfinished thoughts. We had times to reminisce and share laughter and sensitivity. She told us, "The doctor said the cancer is in my brain now." She said it matter-of-factly with the sense of peace she had shown since the beginning of knowing.

Back at our motel, about three A.M., it began to sink in. "I didn't tell her I will miss her." "I didn't tell her how sorry I was that she was going through all of this." My husband said I "would have my chance." I had forgotten that sorrow sometimes comes in waves of pain.

Her son voiced it as, "feeling so alone." I wanted to cry out, but found myself softly weeping in waves that night. We said, "good night" to her earlier and said we would meet her at her home the following day. She was scheduled to travel in the morning. But when we arrived home five hours later, we received a call that she had become much weaker and the team advised that she stay in hospice there. There was no room in hospice back home and her condition warranted more than care in her own home now.

We returned to Rochester the next morning, to find her so weak. Other family and friends arrived that day and the following two days. We were able to talk with her and say all that we had to say and share. I believe everyone did. But even she said she, "Didn't think it would happen so fast." Many, "I love yous," were shared during those hours. How fortunate we were to have her, but this was too soon to see her go. No time was allowed to come to terms with her dark companion. No one saw it coming. Not even her. But in one of her last conversations, (and she was always thinking of those of us around her,) she repeated her one funeral request: "Be sure and have them play Roy Roger's and Dale Evan's tape of "Happy Trails To You." "Don't you think that it is a great 'going out' song?" She was amazing, even then.

January 9, 2012 at 1:50 P.M., with loving family and friends surrounding her, she slept peacefully away to her eternal home. There was so little time to come to terms with her cancer, it strikes indiscriminately.

Now it is up to us.

THE MONTH I GREW UP

Roxanne Wilmes

In 2008, my father in law, John, was diagnosed with a rare cancer. It was invading his sinus/nasal area and the prognosis was not good. We tried everything we could to keep him alive; traditional or not. My Mother-in-law, Geri, heard of some natural juice that was supposed to suppress cancer. I poked around and found out it was the same juice my friend used when she was stage four and she survived. I quickly signed us up and got a huge shipment of what became affectionately known as "Jesus Jungle Juice". John drank it religiously every day, mostly because Geri was not willing to let cancer win. She was determined that he was going to beat this, and she was not going to be a widow. It got pretty rough during the radiation and surgery, but Geri got her way, John beat the cancer and made a full recovery.

Life seemed to be getting back to normal, and John got an all-clear on his screen in September of 2010. We were so relieved, no one could believe that he came back from this horrible strain of cancer, it was like a miracle. But then the shock of reality came on November 2nd when Geri had a sudden heart attack and died in John's arms. They had been married for 52 years and he was absolutely devastated. The next couple of weeks passed with him in a daze, just trying to get along and somehow adjust to Geri's absence.

Exactly four weeks after Geri passed away; John was admitted to the hospital in a state of confusion and reduced motor skills. That was when we learned he had a new cancer. The doctors said it was probably a miniscule dot that was not detected in his last scan. The stress of becoming a widower was too much; he was dying of a broken heart that came in the form of a brain tumor. My husband, Mike, and his brothers, Steve and John, talked over all the options with Big John and the doctors. After learning about hospice and palliative care, we decided to do home hospice care at Steve's house in Maple Grove. Mike and I stayed in a spare bedroom and we took turns with Steve tending to the best patient I've ever seen.

Steve's house was a split level with a living room that looked over the kitchen and dining area. We had a hospital bed and recliner set up with the TV by a big picture window. John joked that he had everything he needed in one room. I spent most days sitting with him in the living room. We watched a little TV. He napped while I crocheted. In the times when he felt up to it we talked. I don't know if it was because he was so lonesome for Geri or if he just felt at peace, but there was calm over John as soon as we moved him in. He spoke often of being anxious to see "The Good Mother" again after more than a month. I teased him that she was probably standing at the gate tapping her foot impatiently. I took advantage of every minute I got to share with him. Whether it was washing his hair or just holding his hand, it meant as much to me as it seemed to mean to him.

John worked for the city of Maple Grove in the road maintenance department. News of his illness traveled quickly through the city. His friends called to inquire about his condition. John told us to make sure there were always cocktails and goodies and everyone was welcome to visit. When he had company upstairs, we could hear the voices as we sat around the dining table. He would tell them he was getting the best care ever. He even joked that if he knew dying was going to be so fun he would have done it sooner. We gave him anything he wanted and enough medicine to help him remain pain free.

As we entered into the second week of home hospice, things got a little tougher. John began to sleep more—in preparation for his long journey. We never woke him to give medicine, but many times we could read the look on his face and judge how much pain meds he needed. When he was up to it, we tried to get as many stories of the old days out of him as we could. Mike went online and found some music the family enjoyed back in the day. A favorite of all of us were the old Roger Miller tunes. We sang and laughed until we cried at the silliness of the lyrics. John explained the newspaper clipping of him as a child with his dogs pulling a sled of hay and shared the old tale of transporting his calf in the backseat of his car! Stories we'll always remember.

The passing days also brought growth to the tumor. It was now like a half of a golf ball extending out of his right temple. People were having a harder time being cheerful, it was hard not to see it and imagine the pain. After all, the other half of that golf ball was pressing into his brain. Talk began to get more serious. The trust and will paperwork was all finalized years ago, so there was no need to worry. John just pleaded with his three sons that they get along, abide by the distributions, and please no fighting. Everyone agreed that was the last thing on anyone's mind. He told us what type of service he wanted and had a hand in planning his "final party". The grim details were handled, no more little things to dwell on.

The priest came to the house to visit with John. I don't know what they discussed; it seemed like a preparation and a lot of praying. He even joked afterward that John taught him a thing or two. That was no surprise to any of us; he was a very wise man. In the final couple of days, he was rarely awake. We had been assured that he could hear us, regardless of whether or not he could see or speak. When our son called to say goodbye to his grandfather, we held the phone to his ear. We saw his eyes move and a tear slowly rolled out. He was listening.

When we knew the time was near, we called all the immediate family over. It was difficult, but goodbyes were said. Mike, John, and I stood at the bedside to reassure him. Occasionally, his eyes would open and stare off to space. We rubbed his arms and held his hands. We told him it was okay to let go, go to The Good Mother, she was waiting. We told him so many times that we loved him, and would see him again someday. His job was done, the kids were grown, and we would all be okay. He looked up again, exhaled his last breath, and went to meet Geri.

SISTER

Mary Van Beusekom

When I heard my sister's voice on the other end of the phone, I was so happy. Because she lived more than 200 miles away and we saw each other only a few times a year, it was always a treat to hear from her. But that day, she did something unprecedented: she asked that my husband pick up the phone so she could talk to both of us together.

Peg was so considerate. She hadn't wanted me to be alone when I heard that my only sister, at age 45, had advanced liver cancer. We had five other siblings, but she was choosing to tell only me because she felt I, as a journalist, was the most able to help her research treatments. Our parents were well in their late 70s, and she didn't want to upset them until she better understood her options and prognosis.

Turns out that she had felt ill for months but had not gone to the doctor until that week, thinking it was just her gallbladder acting up. But she must have suspected it was something far more serious. That year, she, her husband and five kids took a trip to Florida and the Deep South—out of character for a family that was always short on money and liked to stick close to their northern Minnesota home.

Her doctor—when she finally saw her—pressed her hands deep into Peg's abdomen with concern. "It's not your gallbladder," she said. "It's your liver." And then, she left the room.

Even if Peg had seen her doctor earlier, it probably wouldn't have mattered. Cancer cells had likely been growing in her colon for years and, at 45, she was still five years away from getting a routine colonoscopy. Rogue cancer cells from her colon had migrated to her liver and, before two years were up, would invade her lungs as well. My mother's sister had died of liver cancer at the same age, so there was likely some sort of genetic tripwire that I try not to dwell on.

When I think about coming to terms with cancer, I question if anyone really does. It seems to me that, when you have cancer, you spend so much of your limited time fighting it that, by the time it inflicts its final damage, you are too sick to even look up—startled—as it overtakes you. When you are not the one who has cancer, you tend to hope and hope and hope, until you see your sister lying in a recliner, copper-colored skin stretched over her face in a canvas of exhaustion.

So often, death wears a bathrobe. In this case, it was the very warm, plush bathrobe I had given her for Christmas that year. It was March now and, as I placed my three-week-old son in her arms, she whispered, "Beautiful" and then indicated that I should take him because he, at perhaps eight pounds, was too heavy for her atrophied arms.

My mother, horrified with how rapidly Peg had declined since treatment was stopped a few weeks before, fled the house. "Let's go," she said, unable to face saying goodbye. I lingered a moment, then Peg's eyes flickered open, beautiful brown eyes that I knew I was seeing for the last time. "Goodbye, Peg," I said, touching her arm. "I'll see you later."

Peg knew that she was going to die, had seen to it that I received the beautiful Italian cross-stitch picture that had hung on her living room wall for years. Although she coughed relentlessly from the lung cancer, and she had to lie down on my bed often, she carefully painted art deco stencils on the dining room and living room walls of my 1920s bungalow.

After she died, my mother and I lamented that we had none of her jewelry to remember her by. I still think that she meant to give us more but that she, buoyed by the delusions of morphine, thought she had more time than she did.

Up until she got morphine, she had talked freely—if sorrowfully—of her funeral and how she wanted to make sure that there was a funeral luncheon after. She was also grateful that she had 47 years to live. "My life isn't going to be as long as I thought it would be," she said, "but then I think of the little kids who die of cancer, and I realize that I had a long life in comparison." I guess that's a kind of acceptance.

At the funeral that brusque, sunny day in late March, my five brothers were the pallbearers. One of my brothers, a devout Catholic, stashed a small plastic squirt bottle of holy water in his navy blue suit jacket, surreptitiously blessing her casket as they escorted her body from the church. He said that she had made peace with God. I still wonder how he knew that.

And yet, I feel quite sure that I've never come to terms with my sister's death. Recently, after the death of a beloved uncle, I came across a photo in one of his albums. The photo had captured a summer's day, my uncle leaning on a shovel in front of rows of gorgeous zinnias and bachelor's buttons. My mother, sister and I were talking with him. We all looked so happy, oblivious that everyone in that photo except me would soon be dead within the space of eight years.

My mother died of cancer, too: pancreatic cancer from melanoma cells that had probably been circulating in her body for years. Two and a half months after her diagnosis, she was dead in the hospital bed in her living room, her open eyes turned toward the light from the adjoining kitchen. "My mother just died," I told the person at the hospice, whom I'd obviously wakened. "Hello? I said my mother just died."

As my brothers began to arrive at the house, I remember touching my mother's still-warm face and hands, kissing her. Seeing me there, silently sobbing, seven months pregnant with the daughter that would bear my mother's name, one of my brothers pointed at my mother. "This," he said, pausing, "is a blessing." He was referring to the end of her suffering, but I could never see it like that, a blessing. The end of her suffering but just the beginning of ours.

Not long ago, on the anniversary of Peg's death, one of her daughters wrote on Facebook that perhaps it was time to stop being sad when we remember her but to be happy that we had her at all. I try, I do.

But nine years later, while working out at the gym, I see a woman who very much resembles my sister, from her short dark hair and oval face to her patient, deep-set eyes. I happen to glance in the mirror and see that I am smiling. To me, rubbing elbows with the dark companion of death is more like that than any coming to terms. Warmed by a memory, you forget for a moment. Next thing you know, have no sister. One minute you're smiling, the next you're not.

JAMES D. RUSIN, M.D.

I began my cancer journey thirteen and a half years ago, when I developed an unexplained back pain lifting 5 gallons of raw beer. Cancer and death were not remotely considered. When the pain only worsened rather than improve, I went through a medical work up. Modern technology clarified the situation soon enough and I had a new title, Multiple Myeloma patient. My cancer manifested itself with an infiltration and fracture/decomposition of my eighth thoracic vertebrae that generated unrelenting pain that baffled my physicians and tormented me. (I would have preferred to have been baffled.) Early on, I did not have much time to adequately study my new companion. With a prognosis of "three to six months," I was kind of busy.

If I had listened to doctors, I would have been dead three times. My first task was to find a doctor who was not so convinced of my demise. Fortunately, I did find such a physician, who prescribed radiation therapy with the apparently encouraging comment of, "You would not mind five years, would you?" I wanted to ask him if five years was so great, would he like to trade prognoses?

After having my spine irradiated, I was told the cancer had likely spread from the initial site and it would probably return within two years. As there was no treatment at the time, for disseminated multiple myeloma, that would be the end. Like clock work, my cancer reemerged in two years and things looked grim. Fortunately for me, in the two years from the time of my diagnosis, a promising treatment arose using an old drug, Thalidomide, for the treatment of my cancer. Thalidomide and its daughter drugs, along with a bone marrow transplant and lots of love, have given me 13 and a half years of life I had not expected.

Thirteen years of living with my cancer, as well as 30 years of treating cancer patients, has given me plenty of opportunity to study and learn from my companion.

Early on, there was fear. No one lives forever, but, it seemed I had had my "ticket stamped". Dying of a painful cancer, at 48, was not part of my life plan and I did not appreciate the new development. My pain could not be controlled and I was not sleeping. Dying promised some elusive rest. I reviewed the things I worried about, in terms of life, death, and eternity. About the only thing that mattered was my family consisting of a loving wife and four children, none of whom were out of high school. I took solace in the bible verse "You must be willing to give up everything to follow me." I knew then that God would take care of my family. If this cancer was going to kill me, I was ready to die. I believe that is when I started to heal.

Cancer and his close associate, Death, have power over you, if you allow them to. Living successfully with cancer is a matter of balance. It is almost like the kid brother you grew up with that your mother insisted you take with you wherever you went. No matter how much you wanted to be rid of him, you both knew it was not going to happen and he would torment you knowing he could get away with it. And he always did!

The cancer is always in your mental peripheral vision. It hates being ignored. It loves stressing you and it knows your weak spots and when to latch onto your consciousness to wear you down. This is a mental and a physical battle.

Sometimes the pain is manageable. Sometimes it brings you to your knees in tears. You never know if or for how long the current chemotherapy will hold the cancer back? What are the inevitable unpleasant side effects of your new therapy and how will it affect you and your life? What will you have to give up next? How long can you put up with it? What other suffering and indignities are yet to come?

I assume it was unintentional, but cancer taught me some valuable lessons.

I am not afraid of death. Other cultures accept death as part of the circle of life. There is no escaping it so do not waste your time trying.

I am a Christian and we believe our time on this earth is meant to be temporary. I am not a slave to things or money. When death comes, I will miss my family but not much else. I want to believe the world is a little better because I have been here.

I do not dwell on my cancer. It does not define who I am. I have cancer, but, I am too busy living to worry about dying. Death will have to catch me.

I have come to look at other's suffering in a different light. Those who respond to their cancer diagnosis, like deer in the headlights, tend to be those who have gone about their life as if they would live forever. Prior to their diagnosis, they seldom took time to contemplate that life could be different than the life they had been leading. They tend to respond to their cancer diagnosis with anger, looking for someone to blame or at least scream at. Or they give up and turn inward feeling life is unfair and there is nothing they can do. Once the patient has assumed one of these mental postures, I have found it extremely hard to change their mind. I believe either of these responses lessens the likelihood of surviving with your cancer.

I am more patient, especially with those I love and who love me. I know I am not going to live forever. I am grateful for the time I have been given. I feel I have had 13 more years than I expected. I am not about to 'sweat the small stuff'. Being right or being powerful enough to compel someone to do something is not as important as it once was.

I believe stress nourishes my cancer. I want to starve the damn Minnesota thing so I avoid perpetuating stress in my life. I avoid others who are too quick to share their stress. I look for opportunities to laugh and smile. I get great pleasure out of making others laugh and be happy.

Where does this end? I do not know. Goals are now less important to me than 'the trip' and it has been some fantastic trip.

I feel sometimes as if I am in a wrestling match with my cancer. Sometimes he seems to be winning and sometimes I am winning. He is a worthy opponent, but, I want him to know he has been in a fight. No one has blown the whistle yet and until they do, I will continue to live life to the max and try to enjoy every moment of it.

ONE ROSE

A Sibling's Grief

Elaine J. (Lohmeier) Fealy

My mother pulled me by the arm to the casket at the front of the church. I resisted and she squeezed my arm tightly and placed my hand on the body. She spoke very sternly. "Say good-bye to Buddy." My fifteen-year old brother, Roger, had died of cancer. He had been sick for three years.

This body in the coffin weighed only fifty pounds. His hair was snow white. His eyes were sunken back in his head. His cheeks had fallen so far they had carved huge caverns in his face. His fingers were bones barely covered with skin and they were icy cold.

They said he was dead. I didn't believe it. Everyone had said he would get well and come home. My dad bought six grave plots. I thought that meant that more of us were going to die. No one talked about what happened except to say, "Don't talk about it, it makes your mother sad."

I was eleven years old and too scared to ask, too scared to use that word die. It was such a scary word, a sad word, and a final word.

My sister, Vickie, was sixteen and my brother Dick was thirteen. They were old enough to visit my brother in the hospital in the city. The hospital rules said I was too young to visit. I had to be twelve to visit him. I had not seen him for more than a year and one-half when he died.

We lived on a farm near the small town of Braham, Minnesota. My Dad worked in the city and came home on weekends. My Mom stayed in the city to be near my brother. As he became sicker, she stayed away longer.

It wasn't that I didn't ask. I had asked a lot of people if my brother would get well and come home. The well-meaning people from the big church in town said, "God *can* make him well. You just need to pray for him." So I prayed for him to get well.

When my parents were in the city with my brother, my siblings took care of me. They weren't nice to me. They would lock me in the dirt cellar beneath the kitchen floor and put the table on top. There were no lights, no windows and lots of creepy, crawly creatures. At first I was terrified. Sometimes they tied me to a chair and fed me food I hated.

Then I decided it was nicer in the cellar than it was upstairs with them. At eight, I had learned that I was powerless to change things in my life. My sister and brother were stronger. The first couple of times I was locked up, I was terrified. Then from the desperation born out of fear, I made friends with the darkness. I made friends with the crawling creatures that shared my dark, damp hole in the ground.

I knew that I could not continue to get that scared every time they locked me up. When I got scared, they seemed to enjoy it. I could not let them win. I could not let them conquer me. My body was locked up, but my spirit was free. I wrote poems in my mind and put them down on paper later in my room. They were my secret thoughts about fear, anger, loneliness, and death. I would not share them with anyone!

I discovered that if I got really nasty and threatened them they would leave me down there even longer. When I thought they were going to let me out, I screamed through the floor at them. I shouted insults and threats that made them furious. To punish me, they left me there longer, which is just what I wanted. I won a victory by letting them think they were in control.

In the meantime, my brother, Roger, was getting sicker. My parents were fighting more. They were drinking a lot on the weekends they came home. The family was falling apart and no one talked about it.

Life was getting awful. Every time my brother and sister came home from a visit, they were very quiet. They were mean. My mom was sad all the time, and she cried a lot. My dad drank a lot, but hardly talked anymore. I knew something bad was happening, but no one said anything. No one told me my brother would die!

I needed my mother to be home with me! One night I shouted at God, "If he's not going to get better and come home soon, I wish he would just hurry up and die." Three weeks later he died and I thought I had killed him. Didn't God know that I didn't mean what I said? I felt so guilty. How could I ever look my mother in the eyes again? What if she knew that I had told God that I wanted him dead? She would hate me for the rest of my life. She was already so broken that I hoped she would never learn that I had killed him.

They said he was dead. I didn't believe it. Everyone had said he would get well and come home. My dad bought six grave plots. I thought that meant that more of us were going to die like my brother. I worried about who would be next.

The day of the funeral was awful. When my brother left the farm he looked good. He weighed about one hundred pounds. His hair was light brown and curly. I saw him only a few times during the early part of his illness. He didn't look terrible. He was thin and he looked sick, but he still looked like my brother. He had a colostomy. I thought that was gross.

As my hand touched these hands I started to shake all over. It was like touching an electric fence with wet hands. Someone removed me from the coffin as I held tightly onto the rose I had grabbed from his lapel. The rose was the only real thing about that day.

Now the grownups changed their story. They said things like, "God needed another angel in Heaven" and "God needed your brother in Heaven more than here on Earth." Some even said he was better off dead. Grownups could not be trusted or believed. I decided there was no God. If there was a God, he was a terrible, cruel God and I wanted nothing to do with him. He couldn't be trusted either!

I never believed that was my brother, Roger, in that coffin. All memory of my brother left me the day I touched that icy hand. I would always have that one rose. The rose was all I had left, except for the grief. That scary face would haunt for many years.

I still have the rose pressed in my Bible. I remember that day like it was yesterday even though sixty-four years have passed. I have no memory of the childhood we shared. I would always remember that I had wished him dead.

A CANCER NAMED ISLA

Kathy Tate*

My obituary will never read, "She fought a courageous battle with cancer." Still, breast cancer it is. And a *survivor* I'm not. I will die of this cancer one day.

I suspect, in some way, that I knew it would happen. I had bought books about breast cancer for years, glanced through them and tucked them away. Not sure why the interest. Then the day of the diagnosis that left me stumbling about, not quite believing it. Breast cancer. My days turned into nightmares of surgery, chemo, and radiation.

And then, finally, the pronouncement that was I was cancer-free. I whirled through the following year, mostly forgetting the cancer. When an intermittent ache in my arm brought me back to the doctor, I learned that it was a break in the bone from a tumor. An MRI showed that my cancer had metastasized to several bones, including my spine. Some of the bones were broken and the marrow in one had disintegrated, killing that bone. My doctors believed the cancer had been growing for as long as fifteen years. Now I searched for those books: under piles on the steps, in the basement under bowls of potpourri, behind the litter box in the bedroom. I gathered them around me on the floor. Some part of me had known all along that it had begun.

I was numb, I wondered about the metastases. My body and my cancer had obviously co-existed a long time. Bones had been breaking, yet my body had always been able to compensate, and I had never consciously known what was happening. That time of peaceful co-existence was over and I grieved the death and violence inside me.

I sought out others with cancer, I listened to their stories and their talk of hating it and how they planned to fight. I could understand their perspective, but I was neither angry at the cancer, nor did I hate it. I began to feel like an imposter in this group of warriors. I wasn't fighting anything. I certainly didn't like the symptoms or treatments, but this didn't push me into battle. Cancer was a part of me; they were my cells.

Thank God, I had a gentle, kind oncologist who listened. He understood my perspective and never referred to my cancer as a battle to be won. I shared my belief that good, bad, every living being mattered, if there was to be balance in the world. I read to him from books that claimed cancer cells lacked the genetic code to live peacefully with other cells. I spoke with him of the drugs and radiation as a form of behavioral therapy. I wondered aloud if these treatments would help my cancer develop the boundaries needed to co-exist with my other cells.

As the months turned into years, I began to visualize my illness as a recalcitrant cancer-child, one who needed to be taken by the hand and held fast. A rogue child, I christened *ISLA*, the Scottish name for island. Like the Scottish coast, untamed wildness and powerful winds stirred about her. I didn't want to destroy her, I just wanted her to grow still.

But there is no stillness in her. Isla moves on, silently crippling all that she touches. I sense my cells panicking—the destruction that is occurring daily. The surgeries and radiation burns and toxic chemicals they have already endured. I comfort them, quietly assuring them that when it is time we will go together. I picture these wounded cells as children in a scene from the movie, *Exodus,* where the smaller, weaker children in the kibbutz are tied onto the backs of the older ones. They are silently carried over the mountains, into the night to safety.

And then, finally, the pronouncement that I have only months to live. "What have you done, Isla?" I whisper as I sit in the hammock under the maple. Isla watches me in silence. I cringe in pain as I wrap my seared soul in soft blankets, holding it close as I swing back and forth. I tell Isla she mustn't touch.

I wander through these days desperately sad about leaving so soon. I smile as I find surprises on my path and still there is laughter. Confusing, fascinating, soul-aching hours, all moving so quickly. One day soon, it will be time. I look out my window and picture the mountains we will travel, climbing into the night. I will gather up these broken cells and my untouched soul, and we will go. Isla, walking beside us.

NEW TAPESTRY

A SONG

Jane Aas

I wanna laugh so hard it hurts
All I do is cry in bursts
God only knows, what to do

I'm sorry to make you cry
I'll drink the tears softly from your eyes
Truth has no disguise

Chorus:
Oh, I'll wake each morning
Thru the pain
And reach for you
Oh, I'll be brave and honest and true
If you need me to

I lay my naked head on down
Fear takes me as I frown
I stumble, everything is gray

Curtain flaps night light creeps in
A glimmer of moon and morning dew
Familiar, it nourishes me

Bridge: I close my eyes with hope, what will be will be, ooooo

Chorus:
Oh, I'll wake each morning
Thru the pain
And reach for you
Oh, I'll be brave and honest and true
If you need me to

Resting with my love next to me
We fly together timeless and so free
Weaving a new tapestry

Oh, what that will be

oooooo

THE LANGUAGE OF CANCER

Marion Dane Bauer

"This is your cancer," the surgeon said, pointing to a small whitish spot at the edge of the ultrasound film of my breast.

My cancer! I thought. *Who says its mine? I haven't agreed to owning it.*

I had been through all the usual steps to arrive at this appointment in a surgeon's office—and some not so usual ones: the discovery of the lump at the edge of my breast, telling myself it was nothing since I'd always know my breasts were lumpy, getting an overdue mammogram anyway, sighing with relief when the mammogram came back clean, noticing the lump again and pointing it out to my partner, a retired nurse, who packed me off to see our family doctor, another mammogram, an ultra sound, a biopsy, the telephoned report: "Cancer."

And still it felt as though the word had little to do with me.

How could it? Cancer was something that happened to other people, the woman who sat behind me in church, a long-ago aunt whom I'd rarely seen, even a close friend. But not to me. I had always been healthy. Oh, there were issues now and then. Mostly nuisances. The usual inconveniences of aging. Even an occasional scare of some kind that turned out to be nothing serious. But not cancer.

"You know," I said to my partner as we made our way from the surgeon's office, "up until the moment he started talking I fully expected him to say, 'It's all a mistake. You're fine.'"

"Boy," she said, "you sure are a good storyteller, aren't you?" (In my real life, when I'm not sitting in doctors' offices, I write stories for children.)

But however finely-tuned my storytelling ability might be, the word went home with me. A dozen times a day I would pause, if only for a heartbeat, and say to myself, "*Cancer.* I have *cancer*!"

Which brought me to that other thing about cancer, not just naming it but living with it. What am I to do with this cancer growing inside me? Follow the doctor's advice, of course. Have it cut out as an invader, a danger. Accept the recommended radiation treatments with all their attendant ramifications. (By the time the radiologist was through explaining the possible ramifications—my lung impacted, possibly my heart, rib bones made so thin that a sneeze might break them—I signed the necessary paperwork in a hum of denial. What was there to do but sign? What was there to do but deny?)

And what was there to do with this cancer? Fight it? Destroy it? Send it into retreat?

I have long hated the war imagery associated with cancer: invasion, battle, after a long struggle. I don't want to think of my body as invaded. I don't want to think of a marauding enemy occupying *me*. But what else is there?

With my diagnosis in hand, I found myself surrounded by friends who had been in this place before me. Wise and wonderful friends. I asked them for language, a new way of seeing.

One woman suggested the image of weeding a garden, but though I love gardens and love the results of gardens, I am not a gardener. Even my imaginary hands don't want to yank at weeds. And I don't especially want to see my body as weedy.

Another said she thought of her cancer as something dark that needed to come out to be known. I liked that better. But though the darkness was certainly brought out into the light with the surgery, little of the knowing that followed spoke to me. The reports that came back were delivered in numbers and nearly incomprehensible language, and I found nothing of myself in either.

And so, still I struggle to find a way to *see* this cancer, to name it. I can't feel it there. I can't even feel its absence.

"How are you?" everyone asks.

"Fine," I say. "I'm just fine."

How else is there to be? The surgery site is healed, and the first weeks of radiation have brought mostly a disrupted schedule. At least, I'm aware of little else.

I feel an immense tenderness toward my body these days, all of it, even toward the cancer. Even toward *my* cancer. Gone now. Presumably. Do I still have cancer? Will I have it again? Is my body any less mine if the cancer remains or returns?

And I am still without words for what is happening to me, I who live by words.

Maybe it is foolishness on my part to eschew the language of battle. What was it, after all, that the surgeon's skillful hands accomplished except an invasion, a routing of an enemy? What does the radiation achieve, day after day, week after week, except its own killing . . . along with the inevitable collateral damage?

Perhaps, I am being hopelessly romantic, terminally female not to embrace the scouring of this occupying force.

And yet . . . and yet . . . something deeper stirs in me, deeper than any war. It speaks of all that lies hidden so close to my heart. My cancer. My birth. My death.

I was born to die. We were all born to die. It is the inevitable, the only end of all our striving. The gift is to know this truth in time.

In time for what? In time to live. One day, one minute, one breath at a time.

The surgeon has done his good work. The radiologist does hers. And yet I pause from time to time to hold my hands protectively over my wounded breast.

It is my own death I hold so lovingly. I know that. Presumably, not this heartbeat or the next. Perhaps, not even a million heartbeats from now. But my death, all the same, as inevitable as it has always been.

But known now, more clearly known.

And so with new sadness—and a more profound joy—I move into my life.

WILLIAM MCCARTHY

"My wife was diagnosed with breast cancer in 2005. The first poem was written shortly after diagnosis. The second poem was written after surgery. She has been cancer free for nearly seven years."

THE ARRIVAL

We don't know where it came from
but a lump like a small curled worm
has appeared in the white pear fruit
of your right breast.

Is it alien, or some unknown part of you?
Should we set another plate at the table?
Can it be coaxed to leave with love and laughter?

We feed it from "A Fish Called Wanda"
and "Raising Arizona,"
quench its thirst with our tears and
surround it with your children's love.
But in night's dark belly, I strike deals
with gods whose names I had all but forgotten.

DARK COMPANION

It's not like removing a bullet
in the old west, where
the whiskey-soaked doc
drops the lead fragment—
clank— into a silver tray
and says, "Got it.
You're gonna make it
young feller."

This seems more exorcism
than extraction.
When it's over
they wheel you
through sliding glass
doors as somewhere

a clock starts its count
back from five years.

We step into a future
fragile as new lake ice
black water sleeping
beneath us like
a hungry Grendel.
We hold hands
take cautious steps
listen through our feet
for the crack or creak
that might tell us
the moment
he wakes
ready to draw
us under.
But all is silent.

In time our stride smooths
we no longer look down.
I notice how well
our hands fit together
no fumbling as
with a stranger.
Our grip loosens,
the grasp is lighter.

When we pause
my index finger
traces yours out to
where its curved shore
meets the cool lake
smoothness of your
fingernail
following it
to the sharp edge
going over
flowing under
until your finger
closes around mine
and we keep walking.

CANCER...IT'S A GAME CHANGER

Cheryl Stratos

No matter what it is you're fighting or what stage—Cancer is a game changer. You will never leave the same way you arrived. This bad boy comes into my life on September 7th, 2009, the day after I turn 45. My body starts to short-circuit. I feel this strange feeling of numbness all over. A bunch of tests later, they conclude that the numbness is likely caused by the onset of multiple sclerosis (MS). How can this be happening to me? I'm an active, healthy, and never sick chick. I don't even have a regular doctor! Now, I need a neurologist.

My neurologist orders an MRI and finds something "strange" on my liver. "Better get that checked out with your family doctor", he says. CRAP! And so my nightmare begins: Trips to doctors, hospitals and then the PET scan, the final test, the moment of truth. Waiting is the hardest part of the entire process. A recording goes off in the back of my mind, *I have cancer. I don't have cancer. I'm going to die of cancer.* Make it stop!

Suddenly, Pac-Man appears. I start imagining thousands of tiny Pac-Men swimming through my body eating up all the bad cells. I am going to cure myself—mind over matter, yea! And I haven't even been diagnosed yet.

Waiting for that call resembles waiting for the lotto, win big or lose bigger. Then it comes. "Your results are in," POW! "you have cancer!" My body lights up like a Christmas tree, cancer in my lungs, liver, lymph nodes, running all through my uterus. I'm dreaming, surely. But the doctor is still on the other line, and the results are still the same, and I still have cancer.

Biopsy equals pure hell! I lay on a cold iron bed just sedated enough to react to what I am being told by the doctors, trying not to move as they pierce a needle through my liver. By the way, if a doctor says this may hurt be prepared, it is going to hurt like hell! I then hear, "Don't move because we could puncture your lung" suddenly I cannot breathe. It happens! What are the odds?

Next step, naming it, I discover there are thousands of different variations, mutations and scenarios. Did you know it takes two full weeks to do a full pathology on a biopsy?

Twenty-six days later the results are in: **Stage IV Melanoma Cancer**. Is this bad on the scale of cancer? What are my odds? How do I beat this? My brain started spinning and fingers Googling. It's bad. No new, successful melanoma protocol for nearly 15 years. *Don't panic. Stay cool. Have a drink or better yet a shot. There has to be an up side to all this. Medical Marijuana?*

Getting an appointment with an expert or specialist is ridiculous. Two weeks before you can see this guy, four weeks for that guy, and six weeks for some other guy. I could be dead by then! Frustrating.

Turns out newly diagnosed cancer patients need to be investigators. You also need a canceierge someone who can help you navigate the process, my husband Mike, and he is good at it. Emotions aside my new job, Cancer Warrior. Not something you apply for but like it or not, I am a recruit. My husband and I network, analyze and study the best treatment options. We reach out to friends, family and friends of friends. This is the hardest part, admitting I needed help. After much wheeling and dealing, plus some divine intervention I find myself at Memorial Sloan Kettering (MSK), the big kahuna of all cancer centers.

Welcome to MSK—we are waiting in a spa like setting, relaxed and sipping cappuccino. Maybe I am dreaming, was this a hospital? If you have cancer this must be the place to be. I am prepped and questioned by a crew of young doctors. Then I meet the cancer God, we spend three glorious minutes together. I find out my melanoma didn't start as a typical skin irritation or mole—they think it started in my lung. How does someone get "sun" cancer in their lung? Did I leave my mouth open at the beach? The doctor tells me I should consider a clinical trail, as human lab rat. Signing up to be a lab rat is not easy, and it has its challenges, but when your odds suck as bad as mine, you take a chance. I decided to go with it, but reminded myself to expect the unexpected.

Fast-forward five weeks; I am scheduled to start treatment on January, 12, 2010 at MSKCC. I call to confirm my appointment and find out the trial is not approved to start until March— REALLY MARCH! They say I only have 8–10 months! What do I do now? GAME ON!

My husband, Mike, goes from star to superstar. He locks himself in his office and researches like a mad man. The study has been approved in California and limited to 20 people throughout the US. We have to figure out what hospital and who. The telethon begins; getting into a clinical trial and getting treated is not easy. It is a lot like applying for a scholarship in an Ivy League school.

Bingo! A call back from UCLA, few hundred transfers later I get an appointment! I feel like I'm running a marathon to save my life, my competition not other runners but CANCER! And he is one fast bastard. I get my records transferred and find myself meeting with my new doctor in the city of angels. I soon begin my job as the human pincushion at UCLA. All the time thinking *is this REALLY happening to ME?*

I spend five-days in the Ronald Reagan wing at UCLA Ocean view, movie stars. I curse through a series of tests and blood draws. In one day, I'm stuck 52 times with needles. I think I'm in the clear until side effects remind me of the harsh reality. It is all too real now, the high fever, rash, skin peeling off, and sores popping out all over my face. For ten days, I sit in a dark room holding my husband's hand wishing this a troubled dream. I should have stuck with the Pac-Man.

I sleep through most of the summer of 2010. I try to get normal back. But there is no normal when you have cancer. I've been in this clinical trial now for 24 months, and during that time PLX4032 becomes the fastest drug ever approved by the FDA. This magic pill has stopped my cancer from growing. The lights go out on my last PET/CT. I'm one of the "outliers"

There is no "manual" available for surviving cancer. I have learned to think out of the box and get fit for the race of my life. Who knows where the next competition will take me, I have learned to be flexible, appreciative, value each day and enjoy every moment. Some people live 90 years and never understand the importance of this.

I am winning!

ATOSSA SHAFAIE

Cancer happens to everyone else. Until it happens to someone you love. I have never been a bystander, always the one to step up and get it done. "Believe and great things happen", easy to say when you're not in the hot seat. And as always life forces me to see things a different way.

While on a trip to Iran, my mother calls me. "My arm broke." Her arm broke? Getting out of a taxi? Shattered from elbow to shoulder. What causes something like that? Stage IV Neuro-Endocirine Cancer originating in her liver. None of us take it too seriously. What a strange reaction. There are treatments and of course they will work. "Believe and great things happen." Mom would have to stay in Iran until she is well enough to come home. But somewhere my motto fails us. My mother never makes it back. Three months of agonizing bravery, daily challenges to accomplish what we all take for granted, sleep, eat, walk, sit and I say goodbye to a shadow of the woman I've called best friend my entire life. She fades in a hospital bed, her face contorted with tubes leading to machines that keep her alive. She cries one tear, gives me an angry look, and shuts her eyes forever. I go to kiss her head, and feel the lumps beneath her thinning red hair. I wonder if the disease knows it's over. It is done growing. It will die with her.

I love my mother. But she was never one to fight things. She quietly supported everyone around her, let things happen, swallowing the good with the bad whole. I hate the cancer that killed her, the phantom thing that robbed me of the best person I'd ever known. My useless hatred doesn't help anyone. People all over the world still die because of cells that don't know when to stop multiplying. But then when I think I am rid of this "beast," it has something more to teach me.

Three months after I bury my mother, one of my closest friends complains of numbness in her left side. My mother was sixty-three, Cheryl's only forty-five. She is quick to assure there's nothing going on, just a pinched nerve in her neck. It's happened before. We're equestrians. We fall off and get right back on. We're tough. This is nothing.

Skinny, healthy, never sick, always moving Cheryl has Stage IV Metatastic Melanoma. She has a son, a husband, and a business, not to mention her 20 year -old steed, who all depend on her. She doesn't have time for cancer. I watch her become her own advocate, finding trials that save her life. The nay -sayers give her three months, I tell her no way. Somewhere, deep in my core, I know there is another path for her. This is life, this is God, telling her to slow down and smell the roses. That's all. It looks to me as though I'm right. She still comes out to ride with us. She looks a little worn but nothing drastic. Her tests come back telling us all that the tumors shrink, the cancer retreats. It isn't until we travel together that I truly understand how brave this warrior friend of mine is.

Hickstead, a big dressage show in the outskirts of London. Her Australian friend is participating, trying to make the Olympic team. Cheryl really wants to go, but doesn't want to travel alone. I'm in. She walks faster than me in the airport. She seems so full of everything, energy, happiness, life! I'm overweight, and slow compared to her. But then, I start to see the rashes. When she can't hide anymore, she has to come clean that she is nauseous all the time. I have to force her to eat. A minute in the sun and she is tomato red. A cloudy England sun, and 35 spf is still dangerous. She has to wear hats and face covers. People notice. I begin to understand that the hour a day I spend with her is the tip of her cancer ice burg. The heavy mass that she carries around with her beneath the surface is maddeningly colossal.

One particular day, even I'm exhausted. I see she is struggling, but she won't say anything. There is a grand prix scheduled on the other side of the show grounds. We both want to go. I tell her I can't do it. I've got to take a nap. She quietly agrees. We're staying in her friend's camper. We both lie down in unbearably tight quarters and for the first time in my many years of knowing her, Cheryl cries. She tells me she's sorry we missed the show. She says she's so tired of fighting this. She says she's scared and doesn't want to die. I hug her as hard as I can. She is not going to die, I tell her. Not yet. We all die, but this is not how she's going out. She holds on to me with a strength that pulses victory. I repeat my statement, knowing it's true. She is not going to die. She may be exhausted, she may be tired, but she is going to win this. And she has.

It's been three years since they told her she had three months to live. Her tests are still dark, which is apparently good. We meet to go ride, almost every day. But now, I see just how deep she digs in, yoga, meditation, seaweed, pills every day, twice a day, three times a day, funny hats, stares from people, crinkled hair, rashes, and a deep faith that she has too much to live for to let this thing get her, all unite in this tiny woman soaked with a tenacious will to see the sun come up, feel the breeze, ride her horse, raise her son, be a wife to her husband and magnify every wondrous thing everyone else ignores on a daily basis. She is my hero. And I try to remember to tell her every day.

I've never had cancer. I don't know if I ever will. But it has touched my life in ways I never expected. It took a great deal, but it taught me too. I look at Cheryl and I see how life is meant to be lived. One minute at a time, in love, strength, and grace.

WHITE LIES

Donna Luby

As I enter the bedroom, I am filled with apprehension. I know one day soon you will ask me that question I am dreading. Is this the day? Maybe so, and I have no idea what I will say. I've not mastered your art of telling white lies. Little, acceptable lies that on occasion are more convenient, less embarrassing or more kind.

I'm always honest or dishonest, no middle ground. Is it because I haven't lived long enough yet? I am thirty now, I've had four children. One I have already buried. I have buried a marriage, one that I thought would last forever. It seems strange to me that I didn't need those white lies.

You look so ill, Mom, and I know the headaches are getting more and more severe. They are almost violent, so unbearable. How can they be stopped? No medicines seem to help anymore. I no longer notice that you are bald.

You used to hide your head under wigs and makeup. You no longer do that. Your pride is not gone, but the strength to maintain has been taken from you. Your brain tumor that once was in remission has become active. Your surgery, it seems, was only a temporary stop gap.

And now you are terminal. I know that, but no one has told you. I think even the doctors are not comfortable about discussing this with you, and now you are asking me what is wrong. I tell you the doctors say your cancer has returned. You ask me how long you will live. I say I don't know. And when you ask me what I think about everything, I cry from the deepest part of my heart, showing you my tears. I say I love you, and I don't want to lose you.

I am thinking to myself, "Mom, you're only 53. You're young. I'm only 30. I need you. My children need you. You do not say you love me, but I don't need the words. You have spent your life giving love to all your children. Mom, you are so strong."

Even in the process of dying, your strength shows through. You lie back against the pillow. I can tell that there are many thoughts passing through your mind. But you are quiet. You ask me if I have something I need to do. I say I have some dishes I could wash. You tell me I should go do them then. Everything seems so quiet, so still. I leave the bedroom, pulling the door to close behind, but I do not close the door entirely.

In the kitchen, I make the dish water so hot! Hot to help try and shut out the pain that was lumping up in my throat and gripping around my heart. The soapy water burns my hands. Good, let it burn!

I bite my lower lip to silence the sobs. My body shakes as I hold every feeling in. The tears well up in my eyes, streak down my face, and splash into the soapy dishwater.

I think about mom. She knows she has cancer, but how could I take away all of her hope? She has been struggling to survive all of her life and won. Cancer is just one more battle to her. She is a fighter and a survivor. How could I possibly tell her that this is one battle I know she will lose and that I even had a fair idea of how long it might take? I couldn't, and so I lied. It is the only time in my adult life that I have been dishonest with you, mom. I hope you will understand and forgive me. It was a white lie.

Two hours later, mom had a seizure and lapsed into a coma. We were never able to talk again.

HAILSTORMS HAPPEN

Dorothy Sauber

Growing up on a small family farm meant having almost daily contact with disaster. At an early age I was introduced to birthing deaths, bloating deaths, infection, and disease. Cattle, horses, and pigs in my father's pastures and pens lived the Russian roulette life of the farmyard. More than a few of our dogs, cats, and chickens ended up under the wheels of passing milk trucks and farm equipment. Even the healthiest of sheep on the farm might not survive a southern Minnesota ice storm or blizzard, and Minnesota summers were sometimes no more merciful.

The summer I was ten-years-old, my mother, father, and I were seated at the old oak kitchen table when a wind came up so suddenly it rattled the kitchen chimney. Our forks were in midair when the room went dark. The sounds of the storm battering the house, barn, out-buildings, animals, and fields entered the room through the screen door. First came the heavy rain on the tin roofs of the sheds, and then came the beating at the kitchen windows. Hail-stones the size of brass doorknobs pressed down on the farm from all directions. And then, as quickly as it had arrived, the storm moved on, and the darkness was pulled back from the sky.

For the first time in years, my father had a crop in the north fields that promised to cover the October farm mortgage payment. In the time it took us to say noonday grace and fill our plates with meat and potatoes, a mid-July storm stripped all of my father's 80 acres of ripening corn down to stubble.

The storm passed, but there was no air or sound left in the kitchen. After a long look out the window, my father turned and said, "I'm going out to feed the heifers."

Shortly before she died at age forty-seven, Marjorie Williams, a Washington, D.C., journalist and writer of the posthumously edited *The Woman at the Washington Zoo*, asked her doctor why she had gotten liver cancer. The doctor could only tell her, "Lady, you got hit by lightning."

When my friend pressed the oncology resident recently for his theory about how I had gotten lung cancer, he replied, "She just got unlucky." The major suspects had been ruled out. I had never smoked cigarettes, spent time with or around second-hand smoke, lived or grown up playing near an asbestos site, or been employed by a coal mine or nineteenth century textile mill. I've exercised regularly, eaten wisely, aside from the occasional piece of high-end chocolate, and never developed a taste for caffeine or alcohol. I just got unlucky. It is not a surprise that I appear healthy. What is surprising is that I have lung cancer.

Six days after going in for a routine physical to check out why I had suddenly begun to experience shortness of breath, I was told I have stage IV adenocarcinoma, or non-small cell lung cancer. The oncologist, never once losing eye contact with me, said there was no known cure. Any treatment I chose would, at best, only be a means to live a little longer. When I asked for a more precise prognosis, the oncologist laid out the national studies on this sort of cancer: Survival time, on average, is one year after diagnosis. I have since learned that the five-year survival rate of non-small cell lung cancer patients is one percent, or as I wrote later in my journal, "They don't have the guts to say zero."

Since my diagnosis, I have thought often about that mid-July day on the farm. I remember how my father's best crop in years was destroyed while my parents and I sat helpless in our kitchen chairs. I remember walking with my mother out to the edge of the fields and seeing close up what had become of the fall farm payment.

Remembering my father's words and actions that day has helped me cope with my own unexpected loss of a harvest. I used to have illusions of longevity, but now I know that, all along, those illusions were paper kites without wind. Because my grandparents, parents, aunts, uncles, and even cousins grew old, I was lured into thinking I would become a well-ripened member of the Sauber-Devine clan. In fact, when I turned forty-four, I was so confident of a long life that I said to a friend, "I've now lived half of my life."

I can't help but think about all I'll miss by dying sooner rather than later. I had always imagined myself taking my grandchildren, once they were old enough, on trips to places like Budapest, Harare, Dublin, or wherever might fuel their love of the larger world. I'd hoped to see my sons settle into middle age. And I had plenty of plans for the years after retirement from my career as a college teacher. If lists of ideas for research and writing and other projects make for good wallpaper, I have enough to redecorate my own house and my next-door neighbor's yellow bungalow.

My father looked long and hard at his ruined crop before he came to accept what he could not change. I know I can't change my diagnosis of terminal cancer any more than my father could have stopped the hailstones that summer day long ago. But my father did go out to feed the heifers and, like my father, I keep moving, doing what I can to match my wits against what I can't control.

Religious people in the same situation as mine might find comfort in thinking, "Thy will be done." I said, "I've got to get my will done!" For the first few weeks after my diagnosis, I shoveled through jobs that await anyone suddenly faced with a shortened life. I wrote my last will and testament, completed my health care directive, organized my financial accounts where my sons can find them, and researched cremation plans. And along with sorting out my business affairs, I began the process of telling family and friends about my diagnosis. By repeating my cancer story over and over, I began to grasp why the word *cancer* evokes fear and why the word *terminal* brings such grief.

"We understand death for the first time when he puts his hand upon one whom we love," wrote Madame de Stael. But when death puts its hand on our own beloved self, that is another thing altogether. Fear and grief become a suit of clothes the terminally ill can never take off.

I can't say for certain where my father found the fall mortgage money the year of the hailstorm, but most likely he was forced to sell off some or all of the heifers he went out to feed that day. My father thought he was going to have the best corn harvest in years. But he got unlucky. I too have gotten unlucky, but perhaps it is luck enough to have learned at an early age that hailstorms do happen

SO, IT'S CANCER

Lois K. Gibson

September 10, 2000

I lay there, and let the sounds of morning whisper over my still body. The coffee pot started its automatic burp-burble; the newspaper plopped on the rug in front of the door; I heard the click as Larry closed the kitchen door so he wouldn't disturb me.

Now I could hear birds singing their morning song, even though the doors and windows were closed tight. It may be that I didn't really hear them, but rather knew I was hearing them without hearing them. I could hear the rush of the breeze through the leaves of the trees brushing against the window, and I even thought I could hear the leaves turning from green to yellow, as the nights got longer, the days shorter and the year truncated as summer faded away.

I could still count the yellow leaves on the tree outside the bathroom window, just eight yesterday. I knew there would be more when I looked out today. Maybe that's why I was re-luctant to move, to turn, to rise to meet another day.

Or, maybe it was the cancer. Maybe if I lay there, very still, feeling pretty good this morning, when I did get up and out of bed, we would all realize that the cancer wasn't real. It was just another dream; a dark dream, to be sure, but JUST A DREAM.

I rolled over, opened my eyes, reached up and turned off the alarm which had not yet loosed its raucous breep breep. I got out of bed, and realized everything about this morning was real. It is a strange feeling to get up, go about your morning ablutions, get dressed, and feel, that except for the dogging tiredness, there isn't really anything wrong.

I went into the kitchen for breakfast. I had coffee, only one cup these days; my usual ½ bagel with cream cheese and State Fair triple berry jelly; read the newspaper, ready to start another day.

It just isn't the way it was, two weeks ago, at least in my mind. Two weeks ago I was really sick. I had diarrhea, throwing up and I could hardly breathe. But that was OK. I would go the doctor and it would all get straightened out in a hurry. After all, this couldn't be that unusual.

What bothered me the most was trying to catch my breath. But, of course, when you're throwing up all the time, and food that doesn't come up, just goes through you, it would be natural to be short of breath. I never imagined a more sinister scenario.

Today, the wind was really blowing, at first hot, like a desert gale, and then, when it cooled off, the wind blew even harder. For me, this had been a day of waiting. I read, I watered the house plants, I did laundry. I felt useless. My mind wasn't working. I got tired doing nothing. The wind seemed to have blown through me and taken all my strength on some long, endless journey. And more and more leaves turned a dull, early yellow.

Tomorrow, Tuesday, and again on Wednesday there will be lots of tests. Most of them I had never heard of, let alone experienced. We will get the results on Thursday when the Doctor would have a diagnosis and, hopefully, a treatment path that will lead to a complete cure. In the meantime, I pray for the strength, courage and fortitude to face the next two days. I do get the jitters, internally, but I guess that's the way it should be. Anyhow, that's the way it is.

And then the WORD came. I had an especially virulent strain of non-Hodgkins Lymphoma.

Like everyone else, my first thought is "Why me?" and then, my second thought is, "Why not me?" With so many men and women getting cancer, what makes me immune, what makes me so special that I should be spared?

The real question is, "How do you cope with the news? What do you do for yourself?

Can you assist in your recovery, and what can you do for your family, when you realize they are even more traumatized than you, the patient?

I confess, I asked myself these questions, totally unaware of my precarious position, although, I knew it was serious when they drained more than two and a half liters of fluid off my lungs.

My husband knew, my children knew, how serious it was, but I was in extreme denial. I wasn't ready to die; I wasn't going to die. There were so many people, out there, pulling for me, praying for me. Determined not to let them down, I did everything the doctor and nurses said, and followed every instruction as best I could.

When my hair started to fall out, I had my head shaved and ordered a wig. Did you know that a wig is considered a prosthesis, and is covered under medical expenses? I didn't realize that every hair on my body would go; not only eyebrows, but each eyelash, even all my pubic hair.

When I had the energy and courage to look at myself in a mirror, I put on lots of make-up. I scared myself enough. I didn't want to scare anybody else, especially my grandchildren.

I quickly learned that friends are almost as precious as family, in a dire situation.

They bolstered me with cards, letters of encouragement, presents, fruit baskets, and one friend, in particular, knowing I wasn't eating much, brought Godiva chocolates every week, and when he arrived for his weekly visit, checked to make sure I had eaten every one. Of course, I didn't eat all that candy. I shared it with whoever came to visit.

Even though, at one point my white blood cell count was zero, and I was put in the hospital, in isolation, I was determined to justify the dedication of friends and family. I was determined to get well, and I did.

I never believed it was my prayers. I never made any bargains with God. I don't really know why I recovered. I mostly attribute it to the encouragement, the 'never say die' attitude of friends and family.

Diagnosed in Fall 2000, I never thought I would live to celebrate my 75th birthday in 2002, but I did. In appreciation to all those who kept me going in the worst of times, now it was the best of times, and from all across the country, they came to help celebrate; from California, New York, North Carolina, Virginia, Chicago. It was a great party.

After five years of regular visits, and exhaustive check-ups, each time ending with the words, "you're cancer free," in 2007 the doctor said, those magic words, "You're cured."

CAROLYN KLUENDER

Jan. 2012

In her recent summer ritual, Lara is awake at the center of night, climbing from bed, followed by Pixie. She knows her daughter Sabel is silently awake and the three of them make their way down the hall, switching on the kitchen light. The door is opened into the quiet darkness, by the light of an orange lamp at the corner, twelve-year-old Sabel follows four-legged Pixie into the night, barefoot in the summer grass. Pixie disappears into shadows. Fireflies are appearing and disappearing with an ember glow. Unusually warm winds persist, heat lightning noiselessly illuminates the edges of sky above the silhouettes of houses in the cul-de-sac. The fragrant moonflowers seem like white gloves. Underneath a spruce, their white cat emerges, a bright spot in the darkness. They all return to the house and latch the door behind. Lara scoops vanilla ice cream, while moths flutter without rhythm against the windows. Sabel visualizes a nocturnal club, of which all of them, the moths, the raccoons, bats, her pets, and other creatures are members. While Sabel's imagination caused problems at school, over summer break it provides escape. *The Three A.M. Ice Cream Tribe* has now come to order. Without the dad and brother, who are off on a camping trip, they are not just a mother and daughter alone in the house. A caveat of her fantasy world is they have the power to slow down time and even freeze it, so moms breast cancer isn't going to spread any further, they are always going to live in the windy night eating treats, dog and cat will be eternally underfoot.

Time doesn't cease, however, it resumes when they are done licking their spoons and place the bowls in the sink. The kitchen is reclaimed by darkness, another day will come, and then another night, and that is all anybody has.

They all settle back into the comfort of the Queen sized bed, where the street lamp glows beyond the window, listening to wind—wshhh—in the spruce needles, wondering silently if this time, the heat lightning will turn into a storm. Mika and Pixie lie between them, at peace together, large cat and small dog, "Are you comfortable now?" mom hums.

Sabel traces the image of her mother's outline with her eyes, casting each moment into her memory. She is reassured sleeping next to her mother when her father is gone, striving to absorb her mother's goodness.

The quartet nears the threshold of slower, deeper breaths, on a return trip to dreams. Pixie's ears prick up, she's growling low. Might be the disturbing cackle of a raccoon, but Sabel thinks she hears something less organic, she sits up. It sounds like the clatter of someone trying the front door knob. Nobody uses the front door. Curious. Friends and family use the back door. The front door is for strangers. Sabels eyes strain to see her mother, only an outline is visible. Lara does not move, and Pixie, is on all fours, making a low growl, Mika's ears are back against her head. She hears a distinct knock-knock-knock. Pixie lets out one bark, growling as ominously as she can. Keeping still, in the darkness, they wait. After a few moments there's a loud BANG BANG BANG, sending Pixie leaping off the bed towards the door, snarling and barking fiercely, Sabel following, throwing on the hall light, the porch light, shouting—

WHAT DO YOU WANT!?! There is no figure, no outline, no knocker, no interloper to hold accountable. Pixie barks, Sabel searches the scene through the window, her eyes make out no shadows, as if the golem didn't exist.

Unsatisfied, they return to bed, where Mother is wrapped in the sheet like a croissant.

Should I call the police?

No, there is nothing anybody can do about it.

Mother is calm, Sabel puzzles over her lack of fear or fight. The night has turned dreadful. In the past, if they start telling stories, it will help them along.

Lara received her cancer diagnosis at age 37, no stranger to the dark companion. If the intruder is an almost expected, inevitable guest, it still blows like a punch in the gut. After the initial reactions, she finds herself with the heightened senses her grandma used to talk about.

Grandma Eida was the first person she knew to have breast cancer. Lara witnessed these events with her six-year-old eyes, while her own mom Jenny, was twenty-nine with three small children. She lost her mom way too soon, but the grandma had become a grandma, she had seen her children grow up and have families of their own. This memory formed Lara in the times before Breast Cancer became so prolific. In those days, like a shameful malady, it was barely mentioned above a whisper. The word breast, forever associated with life, feeding babies, and meat of chicken, resisted everyday conversation, or dirty word status. Those were the days before pink. The women, Lara, her mother Jenny, and Grandma Eida, handled the subsequent surgeries & treatments with their faith. Now this legacy is passed on to Sabel, too young for children of her own. Many years until she can even have children, Lara realizes, means she may never see her daughter be a mother beyond practicing on the dog and cat.

Opportunity takes the forms of doing for others first, compassion, gratitude for the small things. They accept gracious offerings of neighbors, friends, and family who want nothing more than to rise to the occasion, they bring love and kindness in the form of visits, help, and food, and that is what her cancer has brought.

Somewhere between pity and aloofness is the right answer, but never choose pity. I am grateful for my life, I have a deep appreciation for my family. I have been blessed.

Lara's words hang in the air like cottonwood seeds.

That her mother feels gratitude is a puzzle to young Sabel. The pain of a clumsy intruder, a deadly interloper, is the anti-companion in her mind. Her mothers body is battle-scarred, dark tracks crossing a chest where breasts should have been, a head chestnut curls once crowned, a few strands remain, she wears with more beauty than a wig can provide. Sabel makes a mythical sense of their journey, of Lara as Warrior without armor, and the companions she meets along the way. She snuggles in closer, just a little closer, hoping to absorb some of that goodness and to breathe each others air if only for a little while longer.

LOOK THROUGH THE TEARS

Nancy Roberts

They say your eyes are the windows to your soul.
Seems my body is closing the drapes.
Without my vision, I'm not quite whole,
From this plight I need an escape.
With my mind I still think.
With my hand I still write.
My thoughts and words like a bird take flight.
On a wing and a prayer my words are still scratched out.
My writing is sloppy, but there is no doubt.
That GOD is still there, though my eyes cannot see,
My heart is set on His will for me.
So this is happening, I don't ask why.
My vision is failing, but my eyes can still cry.
Seeing through those tears is my mission and goal.
I feel this fully with my heart and my soul.
No one knows the future, but it only looks dim,
If we lower our eyes and stop looking at HIM!

When that poem was written, I was quite literally, looking through the tears. It was raining outside: as the raindrops washed the earth, tears streamed down my own cheeks. I had recently been diagnosed with Multiple Sclerosis, a disease that has mainly affected my vision. MS affects everyone differently, but at that point, nearly ten years ago, I thought my career as a nurse, my days of driving my kids around, and my ability to read music were all coming to an end...but God has lovingly and patiently taught me to think very differently of my situation. This has been a long journey. I could go into great detail about the etiology, prognosis, challenges, and research that is on-going with MS, but I will pass on that account. MS, like breast cancer, is chronic, is progressive, and has no cure—that's really the "long story short" version. I have learned to live with this disease, but I have also learned to adjust my attitude toward it. So many things have happened during these last ten years since my diagnosis, but I'll stick with just one of my stories that happened shortly after I learned I had MS.

Like I stated before, my main symptom of having Multiple Sclerosis is visual changes. To this day, I have a "blind spot" in the periphery of my vision, that challenges me, but I have learned to live with it. After my diagnosis, I had to take a leave of absence temporarily from my job as an Operating Room Nurse to be treated for this initial MS flare up. During this time, I found it difficult to sit still, so after being treated with steroids, and having my vision improve, I decided that maybe I should learn a bit more about this disease they called MS. On a friend's recommendation, I looked for a book at Barnes and Noble on MS. As I wandered the aisles that contained medical books, I saw many books on multiple topics—menopause, heart disease, eating healthy...not the one I was looking for. However, misfiled in the medical books was what I believe was the book I was meant to find all along, *God is in the Small Stuff—and it all Matters* by Bruce and Stan. I picked up this small devotional book, and started to cry! YES, this was the book I was supposed to read! God was and has been in the "stuff" of MS all along. I purchased this book and started reading it as soon as I got home. It was perfect...or so I thought. I was learning about the Lord and how he cares about what happened in my life, and then...page 152 was not followed by page 153...I looked again...nope...the pages were messed up! First off, I was ecstatic that I could SEE the misprinted pages with my vision being the way it was, but more importantly, I still loved the book! It still had a purpose even with its miss-printed pages. The book was a lot like me. MS caused me to be "miss-printed" if you will, yet I still had a purpose, too. I saved my receipt and returned the next day, not to return the book; no, I loved those miss printed pages. I wanted to get another copy. When I got back to the store the following day with book in hand, I approached the counter and noticed the clerk had fainted! My nursing instincts took over and I immediately rushed around to administer what little assistance I could. As it turned out, the girl was a college student, burning the candle at both ends, had not eaten...well you get it. I didn't do much, but I also realized that I still was useful as a nurse too; MS didn't take that away from me either. The manager of the book store was very kind and let me keep my miss printed version AND gave me a nice discount on a new one as well. Where am I going with all this? Well, I am like the book, miss printed with MS but still very useful. My attitude is a positive one....not every day mind you, I still struggle, but the Lord is with me every step of the way. He had never for one minute left my side. He and I are useful together!

This year for Christmas my daughter gave me a book of "366 poems—One for Every Day of the Year" for Christmas. I read a lovely poem from it for the whole family before Christmas dinner. Everybody got a little teary... My daughter was the one who pointed out this writing contest to me. She goes to school in Duluth and we went out to eat before dropping her off at school. By the way...the book she gave me? Well...it is miss printed... the days do not follow the right order. But that's okay. I'll keep it because out of all the books she could have gotten, this one has special meaning, it's perfectly miss printed.

SURVIVE

Heidi Schauer

Creeping in the shadows of my Friday's happiness, life slithered eighty-one miles down the road and sank its teeth in with one destructive strike. A sentence so powerful my entire body heaved from the impact, "No! No! No!" My jaw dropped, screaming out an ear shattering "my-skin-has-caught-fire-and-I-cannot-escape-the-flame" agony. Words so sharp they plunged through my exterior, secured their truth where it could be felt: "Your dad is dead." I was emotionally paralyzed.

Part of me felt that Lucifer had lunged or God had just turned his head. I wanted to grab the hands of the clock and propel them backward an hour, or two weeks, or three years to when my dad had suffered several strokes while deer hunting. I wanted to be a warrior armed with all the right tools to wage a war and change an outcome. I wanted to wrap my fingers around a neck and pull everything it was attached to so close, and scare it so sincerely, there was no question this was a battle not to begin. But, I couldn't. I had no control.

Spring passed, but my father's departure remained difficult. Wrapped in gold and green flannel I stared at the plaque on my wall: "What you have once enjoyed you can never lose. All that we love deeply becomes a part of us." —Helen Keller, one of my favorites.

"Mama, are you gonna get up?" The electric blue eyes of my four-year-old danced over and her not-so-tiny fingers brushed the side of my face. "I sure love you."

Smiling, I hoped to deny the sting of tears, "I know Doll."

She wrapped her "veggie muscles" around me and sadly I sank. A few memories squeezed out and hearing my sniffle she pulled away, "Missing Grandpa Jim?"

As if beckoned to run interference, her baby brother, who we call "Bubba," burst through the bedroom door pointing and "ahhing" toward the kitchen. Saved by the start of the day, I unwrapped, sat up, and tried to anchor my heels into something solid. With a deep inhale, I dropped the regret of not having lunch "that day" with my dad, and, rolling my shoulders, traveled back the eight months to the present to tackle the task at hand—breakfast.

"Can we have cake?"

The thought of it made me giggle. I love dessert first. "No. A meat sandwich or peanut butter and jelly?" It was easy and what we had.

"Meat and cheese with peanut butter," she said putting the bread on the counter. "Bubba wants that too."

Carrying the sandwiches to a small table, my son pointed with one finger where I should set his. Two sweet babies, how lucky am I? They fought over who would get which plate and which chair was better while I decided it was time for coffee.

Swirling my inch of milk into the caffeine consumption, I felt the sun shining warm on my face. Wouldn't it have been nice to walk through the garden and look for baby birds, or drive through the lakes to scout for "exotics"? But especially in December, and without my dad, those things would not be the same. I swallowed hard.

Struggling, grief circled and I did my best to fend against it. "Mom, someone's at the door."

Marching cup-in-hand, I made my way to the front of the house pushing the damask curtain aside for a peek. It was Auntie Colleen, one of my father's eight siblings. I unlocked the hundred-years of solid protection for a welcomed embrace.

How are you guys?" The hug was immediate. "Thought you might like these," she said pulling out a pile of pictures.

Whirling and thrashing, 2011 had been an unstoppable force. The obstacles were abundant and my dad was not our only family branch suddenly severed. I had battled severe allergies that kept me inside, endured capturing my father's fifty-four-years to share with family and friends, helped hold tight the thread that binds our enormous family purposefully wrapping it around my sister, and rose up after stumbling to the ground to find myself in major foot surgery. After all of that, during the holiday season, my grandpa's time had come. So much for never being given more than you can handle. In my thirty-three-years, I couldn't have imagined.

I grabbed the small stack from my grandpa's house and pushed my mouth to one side biting my inner lip. Alaska. Standing on a hill beneath an amazing tree, my dad married his second wife. He loved it there. The pace was much slower than professional hockey with my mother in Maine, and still, commercial fishing was no piece of cake.

I always wanted a copy of these pictures," I admitted.

I had been to Alaska once in 2001 for the Special Olympic World Winter Games. It changed my life. I had gone with other students, but I could feel my dad there. Oddly, when he was tragically struck I wanted to do the things he had done. To run up the well-known hill in the former Yugoslavia, share a sandwich with a homeless man during Thanksgiving, spend a night at his apartment for the first time, and read the books he had, knowing what parts he liked best. I wanted to smell him—Irish Spring soap and Macho cologne from the dollar store—but, all his clothes had been cleaned. I wanted one of his massive gloves to place his proud, father-of-two, comforting hands in mine. I wanted his triple-extra-large hunter-orange hoodie to wrap his all-encompassing "I-love-you-so-much" arms around me. But, those things could not be achieved.

I drowned what I could with whiskey, regretting the attempt, and buzzed around being busy; but, it didn't dissolve the dark. On several occasions I tilted my head back and slammed my eyes shut pleading, "Please, please, please!" I gasped with all my ability and begged time after time for it not to be true. But it was. My entire body ached as I mourned the loss of a special link in my chain.

I know there will still be challenging days. I will always miss the pile of agates I no longer find outside my door, my dad's one-of-a-kind knock, and his ability to cure just about anything with ice cream. But, as the months move on and pain begins to pass, I find myself capable. Where there once appeared to be an unconquerable distance of darkness, now a flickering flame whispers, "Your journey is not over."

So, I press my pennies into my palms remembering, In God We Trust, and I muster the courage to miss my father with all my might, but begin a new chapter. I wake up each morning, do what I can to plant both my feet firmly on the ground, and take a single step. I choose to survive.

With the clank of a plate joining the others in the sink, I hear "All done Mommy! Can we play outside?" Sipping from my cup, I smile at my aunt wondering if today I will be able to bear taking them to the Como Zoo.

JEAN STEFFENSON

Somehow during the middle of cold, dark nights when the silent world slept, an eerie voice crept through my head…. "Where will you be next year?" "Will you survive?" It asked as fear without any basic rationalization filled my body and made my breath stop. It just went on, "What about your children? Will you see them graduate?" Then, I felt a huge shiver as it whispered, "What happens when you die?"

"Please stop," said my rational side. *Please.* However, my mind raced on the thoughts based on a diagnosis of melanoma. Fear of the unknown had fired through my brain like an engine that couldn't slow down.

How did I know that a dark spot on my face would cause such overpowering thoughts? Once it was removed, I was overjoyed. I had constantly heard, "There's a bug on your face," or "Your make-up has smeared."

"No, I explained it is a spot on my skin."

One medical person actually told me to get a cream that was a skin lightener! Fortunately, the Physician's Assistant wanted it removed.

The hospital is small and an Ear, Nose, and Throat Doctor removed the small patch of skin. I was given instructions on how to keep it clean and how to replace the rather large bandage on my face. I didn't think much about it. I was leaving with my sister, my niece and my daughter for Florida in a couple weeks. I just stayed focused on that thought.

A week later, I answered a phone call from a nurse to inform me that I needed to have more skin removed. The question, "Is it cancer" flew out of my throat. She hesitated. After what appeared to be a long pause, she said, "It's abnormal cell growth."

"That sounds like cancer," I mumbled.

"You need to talk to the Dr. when you come in," she briskly replied and hung up.

The same Ear, Nose, and Throat physician performed the surgery. His friendly demeanor changed when I questioned him about the diagnosis.

"It can kill you if it's not removed," he announced. When he finished, his instructions were to, "Just have your husband check you over for dark spots now and then and you should be okay."

I have a husband who would not notice if I entered a room without a hair on my head. I wasn't really comfortable relying on him to spot a change on my skin.

The summer before this, I had observed a man in his sixties that was our neighbor. He was an extremely fit man and walked by our house frequently. He had been an athlete and he was a retired athletic director. Every ounce of his body looked strong and lean. He had been diagnosed with melanoma a few years ago. In a short time, I noticed that his gait was slower and soon he no longer walked by. He left this world a few weeks after that. His wife was concerned when she heard about my skin cancer. She told me that her husband's recent melanoma stemmed from a mole the size of a pinpoint. Very few people would have noticed it. I found this very frightening. Therefore, I asked my Physician's Assistant to recommend a dermatologist. She recommended a woman in St. Cloud that is located sixty miles from my home. My records were sent.

At my appointment, I was surprised to have a lovely young woman enter and inform me that she was the dermatologist. She looked less than thirty-years-old. She was covered with a mask due to a cold. She met with me briefly. She did a body scan and viewed my face along with the rest of my body under very bright lights. Afterwards, she said that my diagnosis of, "Lentigo maligna" was the same cancer as melanoma but since it had not gone through the skin, they referred to it as lentigo maligna. She infomed me that she had done an entire internship on patients with melanoma. Sometimes, she said patients can go many years with lentigo maligna but it's never a safe call. She told me that in order to give me a prognosis of cancer free with less than 10% chance of it reoccurring, she would need to remove more skin.

The biopsy and surgery afterwards with the ENT specialist had not only caused some pain but constant inquiries. People that did not know me at all asked me about the large bandage on my face. I was so very tired of answering questions that I sent out an email at the school that I work in and explained all about it. However, strangers asked me everywhere I went. Those that had received the email asked me if spots on their own bodies were cancer! (I don't know how I became that qualified!!). If my husband was with me in public, I detected stern glares towards him. They assumed he abused me.

So, I was not excited to have yet another cut on my face but I wanted my best shot at survival. So, I felt that there really wasn't a choice. That's when the eerie voice entered my mind.

I contacted the ENT specialist who had performed the first surgery. I questioned why more skin had not been removed. He complained that dermatologists were "TOO conservative." He said that he would perform another surgery for me. I declined and made an appointment for the dermatologist to perform it.

The lab report after this third time was negative. There was no cancer detected. There was a big enough margin that the dermatologist was comfortable with her prognosis. I continue to need a body scan every six months and I am always relieved when there is not any problem. There is always a little fear but now that I have faced a few dark nights, I know that we should feel joy whenever we have the opportunity.

This past year was a tough one for many in my neighborhood. One woman had a spot on her kidney removed; one was diagnosed with breast cancer, another having gone through breast cancer twice in ten years had her husband diagnosed with esophageal cancer. All of these people monitor their health, eat right, exercise, etc. Everyone had their "dark" moments. Each of them amazed me with their determination and coping skills.

We recently met in a group of twenty-four for a card party. We laughed, joked, snacked and teased each other over our ability (or lack of) as card players. Over a quarter of us there had faced cancer sometime in our lives. Cancer can destroy our bodies in many ways but did not invade our spirits that night. Instead of the dark enemy overcoming us, we rose above it with our ability to continue to enjoy our lives. We have learned that life needs to be celebrated. Smiles, friendship, and laughter can fight the gloomy times and make us realize that we can still have many precious wonderful times left in our lives. Perhaps, we can only know happiness after experiencing some despair. We all hope that the moments of joy in our lives surpass those of pain. It is my wish for all of you.

A CHANGE OF HEARTS

Rosanna Klepper

While I was cleaning up Ma after a particularly nasty and pungent bowel movement, my father paused in her doorway. She said, "Don't you want to help with any of this?"

"No," he said as he turned on his heel and continued down the hallway. Ma began to cry. I challenged him, "Weren't you listening during your vows? In sickness and in health?" I glowered at the now empty doorframe. Just like him not to lift a bloody finger. Let someone else do it. I couldn't believe he was refusing to help. After all, this was his wife. Gagging, I finished up the job, rolled her to the other side, put the diaper underneath her and pulled up the diaper between her legs, fastening it on the sides. After this incident my heart hardened.

A few months later, the doctor wanted dad to go in for a geriatric screening. The doctors discovered he had Parkinson's and probable Alzheimer's. They advised him not to drive. As soon as we got in the car, dad declares, "Well, I don't agree with that."

I yelled at him the whole way home. I was already caring for my bedridden mother and this put me over the top. "The doctors don't just say, 'Don't drive,' for fun, they say it because they mean that you could be dangerous on the road. To yourself and other people. Great, Ma is sick and now I'll have to take care of you. Parkinson's and Alzheimer's? Really? Give me a break. Apparently, God isn't watching. He wants to make my life miserable."

I didn't really feel sorry for him either. I felt sorry for myself.

I call the doctor the next morning. I tell him what dad said. "Let me be the heavy. Your relationship is already strained with him. You can take him over to the rehabilitation center and have his driving tested. They will either say he is fine, or he is okay, but he needs to work on some skills, or, he shouldn't be driving. If they say he can't drive, I can send paperwork to the Secretary of State and they'll revoke his license. That way, the blame will fall on me, not you."

I take dad for the test and he fails. He is mad and I am mad. I now have to drive him everywhere for his doctor appointments, taking time off work.

A speech pathologist, physical therapist and a nurse start coming to the home to see him. I had people coming and going most days, but at least I didn't have to haul him for these appointments. A couple of years passed where his condition was quite stable; then he started having trouble swallowing. It was back to the hospital for another test. He failed it; they put in a g-tube. Now dad could only have cans of liquid food. No more solid foods, not even pureed. My dad was a foodie before we even knew what one was. He delighted in eating. No more cooking where he would whine about the food I made. Now it was just popping open cans and pouring them into the pouch that hung from the IV stand beside the hospital bed.

Ma died and I thought my job would get easier. It didn't.

He tolerated the liquid feedings for about four months. Then he started having trouble with them. He'd throw up because the liquid became too much for his body to handle. The stage four pressure-sores on his heels began to break down more. The nurse started coming two days a week. I was exhausted. I was already worn out when ma died and I didn't have a chance to recover. I resented him for the toll he was taking on me. It seemed it was one thing after another; I couldn't get a break. The doctor cut dad's food down to four cans a day. Mentally, he gets confused but he always knows me.

When I get home from work I walk straight down the hall to dad's room. With the exception of the Wheel of Fortune on in the background, all is quiet from dad's room.

"Hi, Rose. How do you feel?" I ask as I take off my coat.

"Fine."

"I've got to go in the kitchen. Will that be okay with you?"

"Sure, you do whatever you want"

Aurora sits on a chair. I ask her, "How has he been this afternoon?"

"He's been good, no problem."

Relieved, I go prepare my dinner. From the kitchen, I hear Aurora guessing at the puzzles. Silence from dad.

The next morning I am helping Victoria wash dad. I have to roll him toward me so Victoria can wash his backside. Next, we have to get the sling for the Hoyer lift and roll him again to get the sling underneath him. We have it down to a science; our routine is so coordinated and seamless, a ballerina en pointe could not have been as precise. Once we get him into the lift chair, I decide to sing him a song that he used to sing when he was little:

"We're all in our places, with bright, shining faces, good morning to you, good morning to you."

I look at dad. His eyes have brightened and I detect a small smile. I sing it again and he joins me.

"Did you like that?"

"Yes."

Next, I jump around in front of him and make funny faces. Another smile and he's trying to mimic me.

"Silly girl," he says.

I tell him, "Me? Silly? No, I'm a whole lot of fun."

"Silly girl."

As usual, he gets the last word. His eyes light up. I am glad I could make him happy for that brief moment.

His condition worsens. He is down to one can of food a day. I feel like I am starving him. The doctors tell me that if I gave him more food, this would be cruel because he is unable to tolerate more. The chaplain visits and she reads bible verses and the Lord's Prayer.

When the food is cut out, and dad is down to just water, the nurse starts coming three times a week. I ask how long he can survive on just water. He is getting under a cup of water a day. I brush my teeth with more than that. The nurse tells me that people can go on for months on water.

Dad tells me, "I feel wonderful."

I am cheered that he says this. He seems to be holding his own.

Now, when Victoria and I wash up dad in the mornings, when I turn him towards me I get real close to his face and say, "I love you."

He is groggy but he says, "I love you too, Rosie."

I look into his eyes. I can tell he means it and I am so grateful.

SHIFTING ENERGIES

Judy Watson Tiesel

Death is not an option. Yes, Reuel's body has already rejected four chemotherapies since he was diagnosed eight months ago, but our love has always willed its way to life. It will again, I tell myself, watching Reuel in the hospital bed, unsure how heavy the narcotics haze is this morning.

We both greet the oncologist, and as he gives the state-of-the-patient report, I realize he is speaking to me, not my husband. The recognition smacks me: I now captain Reuel's medical care because the pain meds have hijacked him. I swallow a bubble of unease as the oncologist speaks.

"The lymphoma on your husband's upper pelvic bone is voraciously eating through bone and marrow. I think it is time to consider radiation. Also, we are not able to manage his pain. I think radiation will provide some pain relief."

My brain is flooded with competing options. If I choose a reprieve from the intolerable pain, we have to surrender hope of recovery by stem-cell transplantation. How can I possibly make such a decision myself? Throughout our 35 years together, Reuel and I talked over every major decision. He looks at me, his eyes filled with trust.

It's time for me to step up. "Of course," I say with more confidence than I feel. "Let's start the radiation and get him some relief."

Getting the relief creates another ordeal. Yesterday's first trip for radiation treatment required shuffling Reuel from bed to gurney to treatment table, causing unbearable suffering for Reuel and agony for me as I watched helplessly. Today starts with dread of the same, so we strategize together how to get enough medication into him at just the right time to ease the pain before the transfer. By the time the transport team arrives, we have accomplished our goal: Reuel is wearing that slightly sloppy smile that comes with even the briefest relief from pain.

Still, the shift isn't easy. The oncology staff aren't equipped to deal with a 6'4", 195-lb man whose size-13 feet hang over the end of the bed, so we wait again for three more able bodies to move Reuel to the gurney. This is make-or-break time, the cusp between tolerable pain or torture. Reuel closes his eyes and I hold my breath as the aides grab the underlying blanket.

"One, two, three, MOVE."

Reuel's body slides to a smooth stop on the gurney: no jerks, no winces. He opens his eyes, smiles, and gives everyone a thumbs-up signal. The whole room exhales, and it flashes through my awareness how consistently his strong spirit emerges when the pain is held at bay.

I move aside so they can reposition the gurney. As the head swings toward me, Reuel grabs my hand. He looks up at me from his flat pillow while staff bustle around us. Just when the bed driver says, "Ok Mr. Tiesel, let's go," Reuel presses his three middle fingers, one at a time, into my hand and then releases it as he's wheeled out the door.

I whip around and burst into tears.

From deep within himself, Reuel drew on the secret code we had created before we were even engaged, the one we used when sitting in concerts, or church, or other public places where we wanted covert communication. Three fingers, pressed one at a time into whatever part of us was most available: a shoulder during a movie or a back rub, an arm clung to when making our way through a jostling crowd, my swollen belly as he telegraphed his love to me and the baby inside. Each finger communicated a word: "I"—"love"—"you."

I am undone by his love.

Our deep roots of devotion are anchoring his core and protecting his spirit. His lucidity may meander, but his heart and intention are securely fixed to me, the Divine, and our three children. I note as much in the bedside journal my daughter and I have kept as caregivers, a vital resource because our shifts with Reuel seldom overlap.

The next night, however, Marci joins me at the hospital. I use the break to close my eyes in the corner chair. She is delighted to see Reuel's old self, playfully chewing on a straw, chatting with the hand-massage volunteer. Relieved of pain and its accompanying brain fog, he light-heartedly banters with them while the volunteer packs up her lotions.

"I'll see you tomorrow," she says as she leaves.

Reuel waits a few beats, then looks at Marci and whispers, "Won't she be surprised tomorrow!"

"Surprised by what?"

Reuel scoffs. "You know what."

Marci laughs it off as another of his "crazy daddy" moments. A few moments later she notices he's mumbling.

"I have to write out a death notice."

"Do you mean a will, a death notice like a will? What are you thinking, Dad?"

He looks down at the folds of sheet across his legs. "I need the notice because I am going to die tomorrow," he quietly announces.

Marci is appalled. "No, you're not going to die tomorrow, not for many years from now."

He takes that in for a few moments, then looks up at her. "Are you kidding?"

"No, Dad, I'm not kidding. You're not going to die tomorrow."

"Don't joke about something like this!" His eyes well with tears.

"I'd never joke about you dying," she promises, jumping up from her chair to rub his arm, trying to comfort him. He weeps with relief and confusion.

I join her at the bedside, opposite Marci. Our eyes mirror puzzlement about how long he's been holding this belief. I cup his face with my hands since he has no hair for me to stroke.

Sobbing, he says, "I just have to let it in, to accept that I won't be dead tomorrow." His trust in us clashes with his own certainty.

"That's right, you won't be," we simultaneously confirm. I wonder if Marci has a small shadow of suspicion like I do.

He stretches a hand to each of us, and we hold on. Soon we're all crying, at his pain and relief, at our sorrow, at this wondrous and arduous journey we're on. And maybe at the modicum of doubt that can't be entirely erased.

Suddenly Reuel starts frantically pulling the sheet up higher and higher. We are instantly alert, ready for the pain that must be starting to surge. We watch him intently, reading his cues, ready to call the nurse, braced to witness yet another excruciating rush of pain. Then he stops and delicately dabs his eyes with the sheet to dry his tears. Marci and I exhale and burst into laughter.

Marci notes in the journal later: "Our ability to laugh guilt-free at that moment is what makes us members in this sacred and strange care-givers club....I wonder what tomorrow *will* actually bring."

Reuel didn't die that next day. But looking back, I realize that energies were beginning to shift within him. He was accessing a deep knowledge about his remaining time with us, an understanding that we, his family, didn't have and didn't want. We had not yet come to terms with death's certainty.

BLACK DOG

Christopher O. Moore

When your doctor makes a house call, it's time to wonder what's up. For me, it was cancer. A decade later, my mother, and soon after, my father, both were followed home, not by a doctor, but by a companion that would dog them to death.

For months, I'd been noticing telltale signs of something running amok inside me—indigestion, bloating, an occasional tinge of maroon where it didn't belong. But after several blood tests as directed and the labs assuring me it was nothing unusual, I ignored it.

Then one night I ate too many peanuts. Next morning, I woke to gut-wrenching gas pains, cramps that felt as though I was passing Mr. Peanut himself, top hat, spats, monocle and all.

My groans finally compelled my wife to drive me to our small town's hospital, where my general practitioner and neighborhood friend, Dr. John, ordered up a barium enema to see what was going wrong down there. Following the X-rays, I staggered to the car and silently rode home to await the results.

Later that afternoon, Dr. John made the house call. Sitting by my bed, he shared the unnerving news. My colon was plugged with what looked like a tumor, probably cancerous.

Was there a tolling of bells in the background, a hanging of black crepe, a waft of sickeningly sweet funeral flowers? No. I sensed none of those. Just the gaping jaws of a vicious black dog snapping at my heels, and I could hear him, see him and smell him in all his growling glory.

"Ohhhh K", I said to John. "Now what?"

"Well, best thing is to get set for surgery in a couple days."

"Uh huh." Long pause. "What's the prognosis John?"

"Well," he said, "Get ready to spend a lot of time seeing doctors in the near future and beyond."

How far in the beyond? I wondered.

I asked about the time between now and surgery. He suggested an immediate remedy for the anxiety. Scotch. That worked for a while.

I had read plenty of stories about people receiving a death sentence, about the denial, the anger, the bargaining, the acceptance. Maybe not in that order—and weren't there five steps?

No time for any of that, just a trip two days later up the road to a major medical center, meetings with gastrointestinal specialists, surgeons, anesthesiologists, nurses, social workers. A tempest of tests and explanations, anxious looks from loved ones and others. And always in the background crouching in the corner, the specter of my newfound companion, a pointer for now, aiming his muzzle into the dark.

One common question, raised by others than just the medical staff was Why me? How does a 38-year-old, marathon-running, roughage-eating guy like me catch colon cancer? Family history? Not so far. Eat lots of red meat? Not me. Much stress? Of course. Or maybe it was just dumb, unfortunate, miserable luck.

The surgery was the easy part—for me, anyway. I lost a foot or so of colon. My poor loving wife, though she never showed it, nearly lost her mind with worry. But she was elated later when the surgeon told her that it looked like they got all of it and it hadn't spread, as far as he could tell.

Post-op remains a haze. I remember once hearing the doctor and nurse out in the hall discussing my pain medication. The nurse said I'd had enough—the doctor said maybe not. I was rooting for the doctor, remembering how lovely it was to lie there, before the pain had started in again, watching the thermostat slide slowly down the wall. I cheered for morphine and all its many formulations.

I remember the kids visiting, a confusion of relief and anxiety in their faces, the droning pastor pulling for my salvation, the cards from folks I hadn't thought of or they of me in years. And the thoughtful, caring nurses—even the one in a hurry who took me for a walk when it was time to get up and move. Chatting with a coworker, she absent-mindedly dragged me down the hall by my catheter.

Thankfully, Dr. John was wrong about me spending a lot of time in the clutches of medical science. The surgery was nearly thirty years ago, and I've had no chemo, no radiation, just the periodic colonoscopies and a couple clipped polyps. Nothing that many men my age haven't faced.

What I have confronted, though, what continues to be my fearsome companion, sometimes lurking around the corner, sometimes at my heel, is that black dog, a mangy menace that haunts me, now and then, even today. He comes to me unbidden in the strangest hours, sniffing around, looking ready to howl.

It would be many years after my surgery that my parents were diagnosed, first my mother with a breast tumor, then my father with lung cancer. My father waged his battle courageously, as they say in the obituaries. Forging a friendship with Pastor Jack from hospice, he told us he was ready to meet his maker. As they wheeled his remains out of the house, I watched, thankful he had passed as easily as he could make it seem. And once again, I scanned the darkness for the specter that had dogged my past.

Now it's my ninety-one-year-old mother in hospice care. She survived breast cancer but will pass away soon, we're told, drowning in secretions that fill her cancerous lungs. She qualified for hospice months ago but resisted at first, concerned that it was a sure sign of an end nearer than she was ready to accept. However, after being convinced that hospice is not a death sentence, she acquiesced. As advertised, the care has made life more comfortable, both for her and her family. She seems nearly resigned to dying, having been tracked by the shadow of cancer much of her life, starting with her son almost three decades ago.

And I? It's true I have been hounded by a memory that snarls and growls and strains to drag me down, a beast that seems bent on devouring me. Has it changed my life? Are sunsets more technicolorful? Have I traveled to Tahiti? No, not necessarily so.

I envy those who, after close encounters with death, seem to cherish life even more than before. But for me, life has always flashed with moments of wonder and joy, no more so now than before. Thanks to my wife, I love and am loved. She helps me lead a healthy life. I eat well and exercise. I try to forget.

When I take Arlo, our charcoal-gray cockapoo, for walks, I enjoy his company. He's old and doesn't see as well as he used to. At night, as he wanders and sniffs the darkness, I watch him carefully. When he reaches the end of his leash, he almost disappears.

IS THERE ANYTHING FUNNY IN ALL THIS?

Amy Lindgren

I wanted to write a humorous essay on this topic, not out of disrespect, but rather from *deep* respect. Desperately ill people deserve more than pathos; why should they get only half the selection when it comes to emotions? It's like painting a picture with half your paint tubes glued shut.

The problem is that I haven't been desperately ill myself. So attempts at humor seem trivializing. It's not that I don't imagine being ill; just the opposite in fact. I *expect* to be ill. When others say "Why me?" I can only respond by thinking, "Where's mine?" Not because I want the attention or, God help me, the awful disease. But because I can't believe I'm still humming along on borrowed time. My inner dialogue goes something like this:

Illness, I've been expecting you for years, but you've hidden. Hidden from probing fingers on my breasts, invasive tubes in my bottom, finger pricks and blood pressure cuffs. We've searched and searched but we can't find you. If you had made your arrival, I'd be able to include humor in this essay and not look like such an insensitive boob while doing it.

It's probably not such a big loss to be locked out of the humor angle. I mean, really, what's funny about illness? Are there good jokes about throwing up after chemo? Funny stories rooted in hair loss? Get it? *Rooted?* No, maybe not. That lame joke helps to explain the dearth of standup comics riffing on cancer and dementia. Even with plenty of material, it doesn't seem like a very good idea.

Well, okay. If the essay can't involve humor, maybe joy can be a stand-in. Perhaps there could be joy from living without rules, or with new rules. With an illness maybe you can let go of something that has been pulling you back, or take on something you've been putting off. Maybe illness is the great freeing agent.

Or maybe it's just a way to lose all that you've wanted. That doesn't sound much like joy.

So I guess that humor and joy are both out the window. That still leaves wisdom. If I'm sick and nearing my own death, walking arm in arm with illness, my dark-cloaked companion, I want to think that I'll be wiser for my experience. Seeing my death approach, watching my doctors struggle, comforting my family and friends...won't that bring wisdom? Ah, perhaps. But the wisdom will be coming to me as a dying woman. And who's to say I'd be able to impart it to the living? Would anyone even be listening?

That's three down, one to go: After you eliminate humor, joy and wisdom, you're left with irony. If I were to get sick, with my illness accompanying me on one arm, then the other arm would surely be given to irony. The three of us would walk together...sedately? Steadfastly? Myself, I'd like to think we'd progress with some kind of hilarity, but that's because I'm still stuck on the humor theme. Maybe we'd lurch together down the sidewalk like the intro to that old Monkees show, weaving and singing: Hey, hey, we're the illness! People say we monkey around. But we're too busy dyyy-ing to put anybody dowwwnn.

No? Well I could go for something easier instead, like a simple can-can. Just a quick thrusting of our legs in the air, first right, then left, as we lean back from the waist. Now that *would* be ironic, if only because the can-can is something I've never been able to do as a healthy person. What if I could suddenly do it while ill? It reminds me of the old joke: Doctor, I'm so worried. Will I ever be able to play the piano? Yes, if you have this surgery, you should be able to play like Mozart. Good, because I could never play before and I've always wanted to.

Ha ha.

I think I'll have to admit that there's nothing funny about illness. It's messy and painful and frightening to all involved. To be the sick person, to be the one who loves the sick person, to the ones left behind...who has the worst situation? I had a pastor once who insisted that illness was a gift. It's a way for the sick person to draw closer to God. The suffering is even good because it helps to reveal strength and weakness, both good qualities to embrace as Christians.

To which I said, Bullshit.

In my heart, that is. I had a good relationship with this pastor, but even so I reserved words like that for more serious disagreements. But the cleansing properties of extreme illness? I disagreed in silence because I couldn't say for sure. I've been next to illness, helped more than one person on the journey that ends in the ground. When it was my mother, neither of us felt better or stronger as she gasped for air or threw up her dinner or signed herself into the hospital one last time. How was that making us better humans? And what does that theory say about those whose loved ones die in a car crash: Too bad you're not having the cleansing experience that comes from grieving a slow, painful illness?

I guess that's one reason I don't go to church anymore. I seem to have lost the mental agility needed to hold two disparate ideas at once. God loves us but he wants us to die in pain so we can be cleansed. Well, shoot, that clears things up.

Even so, I haven't let go of the whole God thing and I can guarantee I'd come crawling back in a New York minute if I received a diagnosis. God and me, we'd be like this. Inseparable. But me and the pastors of the world? I'd try to get out of that, but if I remember my mother's experience, the pastors and God seem to come as a bundle, like Internet and cable. Even my friend Larry, the ultimate atheist, found himself visited daily by a pastor he had never known or requested when he was lying too helpless in his deathbed to resist. And you know what? He liked the pastor, and he liked the God thing. But he died without telling the rest of us what that meant to him. So we're back to wisdom and how the newly-wise dead person is always taking all the goodies to the grave and leaving the rest of us sucking our thumbs. But he did leave irony behind. If illness was Larry's dark companion, irony was the sidekick that didn't make it into the hearse.

There's no real way to end an essay like this. Is this even an essay? Is there a writing form called "exploration"? Because I think that's what this is. Or maybe, "anticipation," because the specter of illness hangs over all of us, whether healthy, ill or recovering. One last thought: I checked the lyrics on that Monkees song and one of the verses goes, "Anytime or anywhere, just look over your shoulder and we'll be standing there." Is it just me, or does that sound a bit Grim-Reaperish?

KATHLEEN SHEGA

"Just breathe." This was the great advice I was given from a ninety-two-year-old woman who had battled breast cancer earlier in her life. I received this advice while trying to reach her daughter by phone who had also battled breast cancer. I was reaching out for assistance.

Research is the mode I have gone into as an adult when faced with a myriad of health issues whether for myself, children, or family members. Now folks can research just about every-thing on the Internet as it relates to medical issues but in 1998, it was a newer process for me. I had to ask a friend to go on the Internet and she printed what she could find about breast cancer and brought it over. For some reason, information seems to bring me knowledge which for some reason I associate with having more control. However, in some cases less in-formation may be better.

My doctor had recommended a base line mammogram at age thirty-five even though breast cancer did not run in our family. Following his advice, I proceeded. Our family moved to Texas from Minnesota for four years and it was when we returned that I had my second mammogram at age forty. They noticed changes but suggested they monitor the changes for a few months. At my next mammogram, they suggested I see a doctor the next day.

That afternoon, I started phoning women who I knew could assist with information shar-ing and referrals. With three young children, your maternal instincts carry you through things with more effort than you realized was possible.

It is truly a sea of information that surrounds you; today more than in the late 90s. I would compare it to waves of information coming at you. Some days, you can swim through a wave or two. Some days, you may need a surfboard, life preserver or a boat to get through the bigger or numerous waves. The professionals try to assist you as best they can, but often treatment decisions are ultimately left in your hands.

Faith is my foundation—truly. So as I talked with friends or family, I welcomed their offer of prayers. When I was starting this battle with breast cancer, it was the night before the lumpectomy and I felt a wave of calmness come over me. It was wonderful. Unfortunately, I tend to be a worrier by nature and think things through way too far. When this calmness ar-rived, it didn't take me long to realize it was an answer to prayers and to realize things are truly out of my hands.

When I woke up from the lumpectomy, I asked if I could see the African American nurse that had been nice enough to hold my hand in recovery. They told me there wasn't one there. I knew there had been one, but maybe not one that they could see. I remember her vividly. She asked what she could do for me and I asked her to just hold my hand. This was my first visit from an angel that I could see and it has stayed with me.

Through these months of diagnosis and treatment, we had interesting dinner conversa-tions with our children. We were expecting tough questions from the older two but it sur-prised us when our first grader would ask the most honest questions. We encouraged all of them to keep talking with us and asked their school teachers to be alert and willing to assist them if, and when, it might be needed. The youngest wanted to see where I had radiation treatments. So we took them and had milkshakes afterwards. My last treatment was right before Christmas in 1998, the year I turned fourty. Our middle child wrote a book for me as a Christmas present—which made me cry when I realized she had received the message I had been trying to relay. When you have cancer there is only so much you can do and the rest is out of our hands. She had understood that faith was carrying me and us.

The Dark Companion causes many challenges along the way. Students had told the kids on the school bus that I would be dying. So we addressed that straight on. None of us know how long we will live so it is important to live your life well each day.

When our first child was born six weeks early due to toxemia, we were told he might not make it as he was not breathing when born. So once they had him breathing, we had him baptized. That night, I remember vividly praying that if he could live a healthy happy life to let him live, and if not, to please give me the strength to deal with that. It was touch and go for a few days and that preemie is now twenty-seven and has blessed many peoples' lives.

As mentioned earlier, we have had many family medical issues to deal with over the years. I have become astute at researching them and then preparing the related questions to ask the doctors. Prayer is a daily part of my life. The prayers include those I know that need the prayers, as well as those I don't know. I want them to experience the calm in the medical storms and during the tidal waves following.

Survivors deal with this dark companion in various ways. Some volunteer and want to tell their story. Some need time to resurface. Some feel guilt for having survived.

After fourteen years, I thank you for the opportunity to share part of my story. After learning I had breast cancer, the best advice I was given was to "just breathe". My advice to others is to research your alternatives and definitely rely on your faith. You will find supporters in places you were not aware existed.

The National Cancer Institute has great information regarding current best treatments globally for both the patient and doctors. The American Cancer Society provides strong resources as well. I wish you peace in your journey.

SOMETHING OFF MY CHEST

Mara Hart

Thirty years ago, when I was forty-eight, I was diagnosed with breast cancer. I was the collection development librarian at the University of Minnesota, Duluth, living in Superior, Wisconsin with my husband, Ray, and my daughter Jenny, a sophomore in high school. My son, Steve, was a student at University of Wisconsin-Madison. This diagnosis changed my life course entirely, but not in the way I had expected.

As my nurse friend Marion and I sat in her kitchen drinking herbal tea, after telling her of my diagnosis, I asked for the name of a good surgeon. Instead she said to me: "Mara, you've got to get something off your chest. How about Ray?"

She had to be kidding. Ray, my poet husband of thirteen years on whom I depended? Ray, who loved and needed me so much? Of course I loved him too. Or did I? "That's ridiculous," I said. I was confused, and this added to my depression and feelings of helplessness. She gave me the name of a surgeon, and I left.

But I couldn't get her words out of my head.

During a routine physical the week before, my doctor had felt a lump in my right breast. After an aspiration and an x-ray, he phoned with the results: "Well, Mara, it doesn't look good. You'll need to consult a surgeon." Those words had brought me to Marion.

I thought and thought about Marion's words. Might there really be a relationship between Ray and my breast lump? I couldn't see it, and didn't want to see it. I couldn't sleep. My doctor prescribed Lithium.

The surgeon said: "Well, I suppose you already know the bad news. The x-rays clearly show you have a cancerous growth in your right breast, so you'll need a mastectomy. The sooner the better." I was not surprised. *That's* why I had been feeling so depressed and anxious, so powerless, and why my body hurt all over. It seemed only natural. I could scarcely walk around the block alone, and I could not possibly drive our VW station wagon with a stick shift. Since we had had that terrible accident on the Blatnik Bridge, I had a phobia about crossing it. I was, in short, a mess.

We looked at the X-rays together, and he showed me the area of cancer. Yes, there was definitely something there, but I had no way of identifying it. After the operation, he said, I'd be in the hospital for a week, and then home recovering for about a month. The receptionist scheduled surgery for a mastectomy in ten days. On the way out of the office the surgeon said to Ray: "You need to know that she has a life-threatening disease. Be good to her." I felt small and old and gray.

So it was definite. I had cancer, and might not survive. Of course, that knowledge profoundly altered my life view. I saw Marian again, who reiterated—this time more strongly—that I should get Ray off my chest. Should I listen to her? I bought a journal and began to write feverishly in it. How did I want to spend the remainder of my life? What did I wish for my children? I made lists: what was good about my marriage, what was bad? For the first time, I acknowledged that Ray was an alcoholic who at times was violent.

But, with this diagnosis and with Marion's words, something began welling up inside me. My heart was opening up to new possibilities, and reaching down to some determination and self-assertion I hadn't felt in years. Maybe, I *could* change my life. Even though I had never lived alone, maybe I *could*. Maybe I *would* be happier without Ray. I played and played with this intriguing thought, and I came to this conclusion: If I have only a few more years to live, they're going to be as good as possible for my children and for me. I planned a summer trip to Florida with them. And I consulted a lawyer, just in case.

A friend at work suggested I get a second opinion, so I went to the Free Clinic. There the nurse-practioner said "You have to wait twenty-four hours to be sure the biopsy is not a false positive. Remind the surgeon of this." And so I did.

"I won't let you do the biopsy and the mastectomy the same day," I told the surgeon over the phone. "You'll have to schedule the mastectomy later."

"That's nonsense," he said. "The biopsy results take twenty minutes, and you'll still be sedated. It's too risky to have two operations. You have high blood pressure and your system may not be able to handle it." I insisted he re-schedule the mastectomy.

The day before the surgery, I was admitted to St. Luke's Hospital, where I had a chest x-ray, an electrocardiogram, and gave blood that I would need for the mastectomy. I was full of hope and excited about my possible new life. Mother, a former beauty editor, phoned: "Honey, there's an excellent breast reconstruction program here in Atlanta. Come here, and you'll be as good as new."

After surgery, which was at dawn the next morning, back in my hospital room, there was Dr. Tygart leaning over my bed with a thumbs up. "No cancer," he said. "Just your own tissue. In all my twenty years of surgery, this has never happened before."

The next day, instead of the mastectomy, I went home a healed new woman. That night, instead of sleeping with Ray, I slept alone in Stephen's room. At lunch, I told Ray I wanted a separation. Within a few weeks, I filed for divorce, bought a used car, cut my hair, and pierced my ears.

Mother wrote to me: "I have had so many happy days, so many lovely days in my long life. And you will too." She was right. These last thirty years, I have lived my life free, light, and tall. To this day, although the whole experience remains a mystery to me, I am eternally grateful that it happened.

HOUSEKEEPING

Mary Martha Kobus

The housekeeping tips had started a month prior with "Lizzie, come here," where her mother stood in the laundry room, a pile of clothes on one side, the empty machine on the other. "You're going to put the wash on today. You should learn how," and she showed Lizzie, peppering the lesson with, "for tough smells, like your brother's dirty socks, use three caps full of Lysol." Leave baking soda for an hour on the stinky rug where the wet dog napped the day before and vacuum it up to remove the smell; newspapers are best for cleaning windows; spray wood polish on the rag first, never directly on the furniture; use bleach on mildewed grout.

Lizzie imagined it was because she was becoming a woman now; she had had her first period only forty days ago. They were in Lutheran General Hospital, and she had to excuse herself from the doctor appointment to use the bathroom. She saw the spots of blood in her panties for which she had been waiting ever since she read *Are You There God, It's Me, Margaret*, but held off asking her mother for a "modess," that's what they called them, until they had been home awhile because her mother was crying and angry after the doctor told her it was Stage 4. "That's wonderful, Lizzie," she said, and gave her a hug for a little too long as the stain spread to Lizzie's blue jeans.

Despite their busy schedule with the doctors, her mother had managed to find time to show her how to make pot roast (use the pressure cooker, it cuts the cook time down to an hour), Greek chicken (frozen green beans taste just as good as fresh and are a lot less work), spaghetti and meatballs (don't put salt or oil in the water for the pasta—otherwise the sauce will slide right off the noodles), a yellow box cake with white buttercream, and Baker's Chocolate one bowl brownies (always cook them five minutes less than the directions on the box).

Saturday, Lizzie's mother announced they were to make an apple pie. This was the crowning piece of her mother's repertoire, and Lizzie knew that she was only privileged enough to learn this because she was now a woman at twelve years old.

They sat opposite of each other at the cleared kitchen table, two cutting boards, two knives, two bowls for the apples, two sets of measuring cups, measuring spoons, two pie plates, two rolling pins. Her mother coached her through each step. "We're mirror images of each other, see?" said her mother, trying to show Lizzie how to peel an apple's skin with a paring knife. The lesson was just like all the lessons over the years when Lizzie had to mirror her mother: here's how to hold a pen, here's how to sew a stitch. After ten minutes of showing her how to start, Lizzie resolved to use a potato peeler. "I'm left handed," she explained to her mother, "things like this don't come natural to me," the same thing she had said about sewing and good penmanship: it was their routine.

As they measured out the sugar, the brown sugar, the salt, all the dry ingredients that would give the filling that perfect flavor, Lizzie said, "Why don't we put in more brown sugar this time? I like brown sugar better than white."

Her mom paused, holding the measuring cup over the bowl. She considered this question for a moment, then said, "We're always going to want a teaspoon more of this, a half cup more of that. But the proportions are as they are for a reason. Too much cinnamon and you couldn't taste the tartness of the apples; without a pinch of salt you wouldn't notice the ginger. And too much sugar would obscure the apples' own sweetness."

They finished their work by pressing the backs of the tines of their forks into the soft, uncooked crust. When the oven was hot enough they set the pies inside, her mother forcing her to wear oven mitts though they made her hands clumsy, inarticulate.

Normally, they might have retired to the living room where Lizzie would play "Moon River" and "Wouldn't it be Loverly" on the upright, the two of them singing along, pressed together on the piano bench, popping up between songs to lift pieces of tattered sheet music out of the bench for their next number. But Lizzie hadn't played piano in four weeks, since the first round of chemo. Her mom said, "Why don't you lie down for a while. I'll wake you when the buzzer rings." Lizzie nodded and took off the red polka-dotted scarf she had been wearing and padded to the bedroom, hair falling softly from her head like the leaves fell from the trees outside.

When the pies were done, they took them from the oven, and cut into them hastily. "Normally we should let them cool," Lizzie's mother said, "but we don't have time for all that. Besides, we need to test them before your brother and your father get home. Quality control."

She cut into Lizzie's pie first, then her own, making a slice for each of them from each pie. They were identical. "But see?" she asked. "I was right, wasn't I? They come out perfect every time. Just the right amount of everything, Lizzie. Perfect." Lizzie and her mother took eager forks full from each of the pieces, steam rising onto their faces, making their cheeks flush.

Lizzie thought of what her Mother had said about the proportions of ingredients for their pies and a resurgence of anger flooded her. She knew that her mother was teaching her all of this to distract her from the chemo, to make her into a woman, to show Lizzie all the things they wouldn't have time to share as the days were measured in half cups, in teaspoons, in pinches. Where Lizzie wanted a whole cup—no, two cups, five cups, a pound—of time, she had been given three tablespoons full. She was already on her third tablespoon, and she wanted to dip into the bag of time to measure out just one more, but no matter. One day, and soon, her mother would remove one bowl from the cupboard and one paring knife. She would use one rolling pin and one pie plate. There would be no one to mirror.

Instead of telling her mother all she could see now, she held back. She was still tired anyway, and Lizzie didn't want to lash out. All Lizzie could muster was, "Still, I would have *liked* more brown sugar is all."

EMBARKING ON THIS JOURNEY BEYOND SHAME

Patricia A. Gott

"Our words are wiser than we are." —Kathleen Norris

In recent years, much of my mid-forty something life has been preoccupied with meditations on learning how to deal with my illness and the sickness and death of loved ones. I dislike illness, not just as we dislike something on Facebook, but on a much more cogent, visceral level. And yet at the same time, I have had to learn to embrace or at least gradually accept the presence of illness as a regular part of my life. In this embrace, I have felt alone, but paradoxically, I have also felt something akin to triumph in this embrace. Let me share this with you.

Having been diagnosed with ulcerative colitis some twenty years ago, I suffer from occasional depression and intermittent anxiety about it. Many healthy people are unaware of the existence of ulcerative colitis or possess misapprehensions about it and most of my friends and coworkers don't know I have it. Of those who *have* heard of it, some assume that this disease involves some sort of behavioral issue, or that my anxiety is the cause of it—a clear example of blaming the victim, as Susan Sontag notes in *Illness as Metaphor and AIDS and its Metaphors*. For those who do have a glimmer of an idea, most don't fully understand what I deal with on a daily basis, namely the worry about being caught in a compromising position related to not finding and getting to a bathroom in time but also the intensely debilitating intestinal pain associated with ulcerative colitis, pain that some medical professionals have anecdotally compared to the pangs of childbirth. However, it's not the illness itself or the misapprehensions about it that worry me, it's the feelings of shame that my disease sometimes causes me to feel.

The shame emerges in part from the seclusion I enforce on myself as a way of decompressing from a sometimes lonely and stressful job and life. When I venture out, I usually have to "case the joint," so to speak, to determine where the bathrooms are located. When those bathrooms don't materialize, physical mayhem often ensues. And though I'm naturally a morning person, I've had to rearrange my teaching schedule to free up my mornings for sufficient time for dozens of bathroom visits. The physical discomfort is discouraging, but even more thornily complicated is the process of fear and of figuring out whom to confide in. Who can I show what I'm dealing with when neither I nor medical science seems to know how to help heal me completely or alleviate my shame?

I have fought feeling ashamed at having such a highly personal, painful and self-esteem-dashing illness. In the fighting, the anxiety sometimes becomes extreme. I know that I should locate healthy strategies for dealing with my illness and the complications it brings, and sometimes I am successful at doing this. However, if I am honest with myself, the truth is that often I am not. Even more challenging is the idea that I wasn't raised in an environment where I felt comfortable asking for help or talking about my difficulties. But I am learning to do so every day now. Although I am learning to talk candidly with others about their illnesses and even my own, I am not sure I ever have let anyone inside fully.

I do derive some small comfort in knowing I am neither alone nor is my situation anything unique. I witnessed my grandmother reduced to a fractured and miniaturized version of her formerly strong framed self after a devastating bout of untreated breast cancer that metastasized into bone cancer, a disease so destructive to her body that she looked as emaciated as an Auschwitz inmate. My mother, dealing with Parkinson's disease, previously battled two rounds of breast cancer as she followed in the steps of her mother and sister, both of whom also had breast cancer. Breast cancer sometimes seems like my family legacy. Close friends have departed from this physical world lacerated by a variety of ailments, including my high school friend, a gifted actor who succumbed to HIV-related complications, and a whip-smart graduate school boyfriend, who, Keats-like, was a mere twenty-five years old when he died suddenly across the country and quite alone at the time. After Andy's unexpected death, it took a long time for me to talk about the pain of others' suffering and also to talk about my own.

One lesson that I am still learning is how vital it is to reach out to others to ask for help with the healing process, no matter where we're at with it. One new friend whom I'll call Leslie is a survivor of ovarian cancer. I had no way of knowing that Leslie had dealt with cancer, or knowing that she would help me with my own illness when I met her, but she has. I talked to her about the grief I felt facing my mother's Parkinson's disease. A truly caring and beautiful person, she offered up some thoughts about the process of trying to connect to others about their struggles with illness. While reading Anne Lamott's *Traveling Mercies*, my friend put forth an idea paraphrased from Lamott, something I responded to mightily. She notes, "It is also good to reach out to others because we cannot stay alone and be well." This helped me to move beyond my shame and learn that, if I spoke up about my illness, I might be helping someone feel better about their situation. In revealing my vulnerable self, I have the chance to help a friend as we leave some of our shame behind.

In reflecting upon this topic, I had to overcome my own prejudice related to illness as well as overcome my shame at talking about something so private and so achingly personal. Sontag observes that, "... a surprisingly large number of people with cancer find themselves being shunned by relatives and friends and are the object of practices of decontamination by members of their household, as if cancer, like TB, were an infectious disease." Here Sontag highlights a disturbing response to a sad issue, yes. Let's face it—illness is a downer. No one likes being around someone who talks constantly about their aches and pains. In fact, I often don't want to be *around myself* when I'm obsessed with my aches and the mental blocks that often come with them! But as I have confronted the fact that I am a chronically ill adult woman, I have learned to listen more closely to others as well as the illness itself. And in learning to listen to the process my body is going through experiencing illness and recovering from it, I have learned to begin to embrace the idea that both my ill and healthy selves combine to make up the whole of me, even though neither one does not define *every* part of me. I no longer experience regret about my frequent meditation on illness.

And so, how do we go about feeling better—for at least a few moments and then perhaps days and months—even though we don't feel well much of the time? As the Buddha reminds us, life is a continual experience of suffering; as we suffer, perhaps we can take a message from Alcoholics Anonymous and other groups designed to help us confront our reality head on: We keep going, one foot in front of the next, one day at a time, even though we want nothing more than to give up the ghost. As Theodore Roethke writes in his lovely lyric poem, *I Knew a Woman*: "We learn by going where we have to go."

At times, it feels like nearly everyone I know is personally dealing with a serious affliction or helping a loved one deal with one or more chronic illnesses, so it makes sense that this issue is at the forefront of my forty-something brain. Our challenge as ill persons and those who wish to help them is to see with new eyes, seek fresh answers and develop honest coping strategies to heal us individually and collectively as we embark on our passages for full and shame-free lives.

Works Cited

Lamott, Anne. *Traveling Mercies.* Anchor Books, 2000.
Norris, Kathleen. *Amazing Grace.* Riverhead Books, 1999.
Roethke, Theodore. "I Knew a Woman." *Collected Poems of Theodore Roethke.* Double-day, 1954.
Sontag, Susan. *Illness as Metaphor and AIDS as its Metaphor.* Picador, 2001. http://www.susansontag.com/SusanSontag/books/illnessAsMetaphor.shtml

LINDSAY LEE JOHNSON

Our paths crossed in the garden. Beyond a shadowy glimpse from the corner of my eye, the merest suggestion of movement, I never really saw my assailant. But feel it, I surely did— a sting sharp enough to cause me to interrupt my planting. I pulled off my gardening gloves to inspect. There, on the inside of my left forearm, about an inch below the elbow, were two miniscule red dots. An insect bite of some kind, a mere springtime-in-the-flower-bed-annoyance, I assumed. The well-armed little sniper had disappeared, back under one of the mossy stepping stones, most likely, but I didn't want to risk another encounter. I headed indoors in search of anti-itch cream, blessedly unaware that the unstoppable venom of a brown spider was surging through my body, re-setting the course of my life from health to incapacity.

By the next day, the affected site was fiery red, painful as well as itchy, and enlarging. I applied an antibiotic cream to the area, covered it with a band-aid, and tried not to scratch. Another day later, my entire forearm had become a hot, red balloon. The bite was obviously infected, and the skin around it seemed to be collapsing into a whitish ooze. On top of that, I had developed a crushing headache; I couldn't move my neck without sending fireworks of pain up and down my spine; and I couldn't stop vomiting. Obviously, over-the-counter remedies weren't enough.

The first doctor was clearly alarmed at what he saw; he didn't have to be told that he was looking at the work of a venomous spider. *I* was alarmed to learn that the tiny amount of poison injected into my arm by that creature was not only eating away my flesh, it was spreading throughout all my bodily systems, aiming for total annihilation. Mother Nature had endowed this eight-legged mini-ninja with out-sized defense capabilities, and I'd become its unwitting target.

By this time, I was too ill to think clearly or to speak. With my husband and two adult daughters, both nurses, at my side to ask the necessary questions and make the appropriate decisions, I willingly relinquished control of my physical self. I closed my eyes, submerged in pain.

Immediate surgery was required to remove the suppurating tissue around the initial wound, and I was started on massive doses of antibiotics and powerful pain medication. Then I was transferred by ambulance to a larger metropolitan hospital, where a full spectrum of medical specialists was waiting—neurologists, radiologists, hematologists, infection control specialists—ready to do battle on my behalf.

Battle they did, with every test imaginable—blood work-ups, CAT-scans, MRIs, a spinal tap and blood patch. After several delirious days, with the systemic infection finally responding to treatment, a neurologist gave me the long list of diseases that had been ruled out, including meningitis, encephalitis, and flesh-eating ebola, along with a host of other rare and terrible things. Even though the doctors hadn't been able to come up with a definitive diagnosis, they believed that whatever unidentified pathogen had invaded my body as a result of my arachnoid assault, it wasn't going to be fatal in the short run. Still, the creature had left its calling card, as if to say, *Don't forget me. This is only the beginning.*

Indeed, that frightening episode led to a cascade of insidious health issues, most of the auto-immune variety, including a desiccated thyroid. A compromised central nervous system left me with permanent neurological deficits; bouts of unpredictable vertigo; headaches; debilitating fatigue; mental fog; and lupus-like skin lesions. Medications and other therapies have helped with some of the symptoms, but it's become clear over time that I'm traveling a one-way path, a downward spiral, with illness. Chronic, progressive illness.

Many afflicted people speak of *fighting* a disease. For them, the courageous warrior metaphor is inspiring and helpful. While I believe in participating in my treatment as an educated and involved advocate, I prefer to think of the medical professionals as my representatives in the ring, wrestling with my antagonists. I admit that on my worst days, I feel resentful. Victimized by a spider, like a character in a nursery rhyme turned horror story—how absurd!

On a deeper level, I see my primary role as *living with* illness, with an appreciation of my body and spirit as distinct and separate from the illness. I try not to demonize the illness itself. Even though this uninvited guest ravages my body as it must, according to the immutable laws of nature, it doesn't hate me. In truth, it functions as a constant monitor of my physical condition offering warning signals, such as fever or pain, to guide my behavior, reminding me what my body needs as opposed to what I may want.

Limitations are hard to accept, but I've learned, repeatedly, that accommodation to the demands of this ever-present companion is the best option. Whenever I try to do things the way I used to—babysitting grandchildren during the day, going out to dinner with friends in the evening—I feel the hand of my invisible guardian holding me back, as if from a cliff. Biking, or skiing? House cleaning? Walking the mall? I hear the cautionary whisper, *Consider the cost. The price may be too great.* It's true; one activity in a day is my limit. Next Tuesday—either meet with the library committee, or go to the beauty salon. Not both. And always, I must schedule time for rest and recovery from even these minor exertions.

Of course, I miss many of the activities I used to enjoy, especially traveling. I mourn the loss of the life I used to lead. Fortunately, I have supportive family members and friends. Also, my contemplative nature has eased the process of adjusting. I've never required the constant stimulation of a jam-packed calendar; in my world—before, as well as since, the arrival of illness—solitude is a close cousin of contentment, and merely distant kin to loneliness. Thus, it seems natural to me that railing against my new reality only saps what little physical and mental energy I'm allotted each day. How much better it is to befriend this entity, my dark companion, to heed its advice, like that of a faithful nurse whose goal is to protect my health and prolong my life.

For me, acceptance of the disease process isn't giving up or giving in to defeat. It's a matter of rising above the corporeal fray by means of a chosen attitude of serenity. In this way, I will continue to live my days in peace, holding the hand of my abiding angel, whistling together in the dark, until the last dance is over.

AMY PADDEN

Death comes with the banshee's scream, a primordial sound that slides down your spine and leaves you shaken and chilled. The sound makes you look furtively over your shoulder for her dark hand waiting to see who she will take away. The scream is sudden, abrupt and brings an immediate death. Yet when the Dark Companion arrives, he is more subtle, worming his way into your life. Both eventually take away a loved one but the Dark Companion does it slowly, upheaving your life in inches until Death finally comes.

The Dark Companion knocks on your door day or night, oblivious to what is going on in your life. You may not notice the exact moment the Dark Companion arrives, he is sometimes stealthy and swoops in like an owl in prowl. Yet his presence heralds a new chapter of your life and alters your legacy for there are some illnesses that chicken soup cannot cure and some illnesses that become who you are. These are the illnesses that stay more than three days and begin to stink like fish and family who remain in one's house too long. The Dark Companion brings this life changing illness to you uninvited and unreturnable.

The diagnosis of an illness leaves one in a cloudy murk; a foggy void that makes everything feel hard. The things that used to matter don't anymore as the Dark Companion envelops you, pushing everything else far away. The illness becomes the only real thing in your life and, at that, it is a "slipperingly" difficult thing to grasp and understand. The Dark Companion brings a slow, desperate rage that surprises you during the moments when you are not too busy and have stopped and can finally think.

Life does not have the same meaning once the Dark Companion enters. Your goals no longer seem important because now simply living life "normally" becomes an all one can think about. For now, you need to live a lifetime's worth of memories into a very finite amount of time. That's what makes his arrival so hard to bear; your lifetime now has an expiration date. Everything is no longer possible. To feel one's mortality and be limited in one's potential is a hard pill to swallow.

And yet, the Dark Companion's arrival brings a new sense of clarity to your life. He helps you see what really matters and gives you an opportunity to accomplish that which is important. That which is necessary to make your life feel complete and full. One's life has been made finite but it now has an urgency and motivation to accomplish the experiences that are meaningful and will define their life. The Dark Companion is an unwelcome visitor but his presence brings a focus and fire to one's life and a chance to truly shape the life which so many take for granted.

Life gets busy when the Dark Companion arrives. So much to do and one hopes that what you have accomplished and created during your life will leave enough memories to all whose lives you've touched so that you are remembered for all the things you did and not for the illness that dominated your final time. As memories fade, you hope to stay relevant and remain important. It is so essential that people remember you and not have them forget who you were and what you were to them. The Dark Companion's arrival threatens your legacy for when the Dark Companion finally takes you, what is left? What legacy will you leave behind? To create a legacy that will sustain those that love you becomes crucial and an all-consuming quest as you struggle against what the Dark Companion's arrival means to your life.

When the Dark Companion comes, there is no return policy, simply the hope that he's come to the wrong place, the doctors have been wrong and he will disappear as quietly as he came. The lucky ones see the Dark Companion slip away; a quiet divorce that leaves its undeniable mark on your life but also leaves you safe. That hope sustains you and drives you to fight making every moment of your life mean something and not complacently living but living to the fullest.

Once you learn to cope with the arrival of the Dark Companion, you get to where you forget his constant presence. Until something new makes you remember how different your life has become and how difficult your coping has made everything for you. Would it be easier to cope if the Dark Companion had arrived suddenly like Death? Is what makes the Dark Companion's presence so onerous and distasteful is that it marks you for Death? The uncertainty of the Dark Companion means you never get complacent but simply develop new routines and create memories to last forever, not focusing on what is coming but on what you can make of every moment.

The Dark Companion's arrival makes you a hero. You fight for every moment and experience, putting others first by living your time for them and giving them everything you can before you are gone. The Dark Companion makes this simple act of living a battle and his arrival makes you fight courageously to be remembered for whom you are and what you stand for and not for the shadow the Dark Companion throws onto your life and legacy. His arrival doesn't define who you are but gives your life a clear definition and focus as you create your own legacy.

THE TERRORIST AND HOPE

Mary Amundsen

The terrorist has a strangle hold on my family again. Does the terrorist have a travel agent? Does the travel agent use a genetic source or an environmental agent? Is that why cancer is insinuating its cells into our family again? Your presence brings us to our knees. Terrified, we become paralyzed in our own defense. So we call in the experts, those who have scanners, knives, nuclear weapons and poison liquids. They will find you hiding out in dark caves, sending messengers to distant cells to cause more destruction, attacking when we least expect you. You have many names, many faces, insidious ways.

The world spins like a top gone crazy, wobbling, falling off the edge. A ringing of the phone and my son saying his daughter, age 15, just had a chest x-ray showing multiple tumors and possible diagnosis of Hodgkin's lymphoma. Why does the terrorist need to invade children? Why is it happening in my family again? We paid our dues many times over.

The doctor becomes our travel agent. The map is explained and the journey to the possible destination of a cancer free life is begun. Along the way are many players: pathologists, radiologists, surgeons, oncologists, nurses, family and friends. The major player is the patient— the person with cancer who has an altered body image, loses hair, throws up, endures pain, and tries to smile when asked that repetitive question— "how are you feeling?"

It's three A.M. That time when fear pounces on my head, jogs into my brain and forces my eyelids open until daybreak. The splinter of fear is harder to dislodge when I watch a loved one endure the cancer treatment rather than going through the treatment myself. When I had a breast lumpectomy and radiation I felt like I was actively participating in my journey. Watching and listening to my young daughter struggle with ovarian cancer treatment caused the fear monster to invade my sleep for years. Coaching my husband to continue his radiation for the sinus cancer gave me a purpose, at least during those weeks of treatment. Then there was the shock of another young female family member with bladder cancer. And now, now I have to watch a beloved grandchild do all this again. Where in the dark of night do I find the sliver of light called hope?

Despair is dark and all consuming. It smothers hope and monopolizes thinking until I begin to take charge. Along with the medical team as the travel agent, I can take charge of my outlook and response on this latest journey. Fear is my companion but surrounding myself with positive and supportive others delegates fear to the back of the room. It was the family members and friends from many parts of my life who kept me and the other cancer survivors hopeful as we trudged through the morass of treatments. The human connection means we matter to others and that they will be there regardless of how we look, sound or act in the good and bad days. That is the glue for that glimmer of hope. Their unflagging support is the critical element required with a cancer diagnosis.

My first response with all of these diagnoses was to call someone, a friend, my brother, my children, my husband. I needed to express that fear, outrage and overwhelming sadness. I needed to feel the unwavering support of another human, a person who knew my history but also knew I somehow would come to terms with this new family crisis. When it happens to the young family members, I rage at the universe that it should be me. I've had many years of life and it isn't fair because they haven't.

But that is one of those out of control elements and so I draw on my support to find the courage and strength to accompany another loved one through the maze of cancer treatment.

I remember so vividly the night after my young daughter was diagnosed with ovarian cancer. I had come to take care of her two young boys and so was thousands of miles from my home. Her cancer had spread outside the ovary and her surgery removed all of her reproductive organs. The surgeon was devastated by the extent of the spread. That night, I couldn't stop crying which was very unusual for me. I became desperate because I needed to be strong for my daughter and son-in-law and able to care for her little boys. As the hours went by, I tried every relaxation, meditation and thought stopping exercise I could remember. Finally, I started to quietly sing the children's meditation from my church— "may peace surround you, may love surround you, as you go on your way." By repeating that over and over and imaging the arms of my congregation around me, I was able to get a few hours sleep. It was that deep connection with others through our common spiritual path that sustained me during those difficult days.

Since then, I realize when that dark terrorist invades my family I need to feel the human and spiritual strength my family and friends offer. No words can take away the fear and anxiety but a touch or a listening presence helps get me through the sleepless nights and trying days. The diagnosis of dementia in my husband was even more devastating than his cancer diagnosis had been. As a nurse, I knew what the future of a dementia diagnosis would bring and that I would have to use all my coping skills plus really lean on family and friends. Ultimately, we travel the path alone whether as the patient or family member. Through the years, I have learned what I need to keep myself steady on that path and although it may not be the same for everyone the connection with others who care is the catalyst for hope.

MY DAUGHTER KELLY

Mary Jo McCarthy

It was a perfect summer day in July at our lake home. The sky was clear, azure blue with just the right amount of puffy clouds lazily drifting by. My granddaughter, Michaela, and I sat on the sun porch, playing her favorite board game. The telephone rang. It was my daughter, Kelly, saying that she and her husband, John, would come early the next day to pick up Michaela. I asked if she could stay a few days longer, but the tone in Kelly's voice, brought a sudden chill to my heart. She took a deep breath and began, "Mom, I found a lump in my breast and the tests just came back. It's cancer." We were both silent for a long moment. It seemed an eternity until she spoke: "We want to tell Michaela the news. Can you keep things normal until we get there?" I found my voice finally. "Yes, Honey, I wish you were here right now." We spoke briefly, then, I hung up the phone, fully aware that Michaela was just a few feet away from me. That afternoon was a blur of forced normalcy for my husband, Tim and me. When Michaela was safely asleep, we were finally able to let the tears flow, as we held each other in disbelief.

Later that night, as I lay in bed, unsuccessful at sleep, I found myself drifting back in time, thirty-eight years earlier to be exact. I was in the hospital maternity wing, just a new mother of several hours, holding my precious daughter, Kelly, for the first time, her small, perfect head peeking out from the receiving blanket, completely smooth without a single hair.

As I gazed down at her, an overwhelming feeling swept over me, a strong feeling of love that I had never felt before; only the two of us, gazing into each other's eyes. Suddenly, the nurse came to return her to the nursery and I protested. She spoke gently, "You need rest. I'll be back with her in the morning for her feeding."

I tried unsuccessfully to settle down. Didn't the nurse understand that I would not sleep a wink tonight until I planned her entire life, or at least the first few years? Reminiscing, I remembered that I always knew her name would be Kelly. I had practiced writing it in senior class study hall, over and over in my notebook. That night, I imagined her first birthday party, what style her hair would be, where she would go to grade school, high school and college. Lastly, I pictured her in her wedding gown, walking down the aisle, then leaving with her bridegroom for a honeymoon to Disneyworld. I fell asleep.

What I didn't plan on was cancer. Does anyone ever imagine that? When Kelly arrived with John at our home that next afternoon, my husband and I listened with full hearts as they explained the awful reality to Michaela, who was eleven years old. She flung herself into their arms and cried, "Mommy, I don't want you to die!" We quietly left them on the porch to talk and hug.

Since that day in July, of 2009, we all became accustomed to a new way of life: a life of appointments, tests, chemotherapy, devastating side effects and doctors cautiously optimistic reports.

Then, miraculously, something else began to take place. Kelly grew stronger than ever! Her attitude was positive and upbeat. When her hair disappeared, she opted to wear baseball caps and even decorated them to match her outfits. She was a high-school career counselor and wanted to be a cheery and positive role model for her students. There was a tremendous outpouring of encouragement from friends, colleagues and family; even strangers joined in with their support, arriving at her doorstep with fragrant flowers, cards and gifts of loving-kindness. We organized a "pink envelope" ministry, where get-well wishes arrived almost daily to bring her encouragement. It was amazing to behold. Kelly's faith, became even stronger, a powerhouse of true belief that blossomed anew as she progressed through her treatments. Her bilateral breast surgery soon followed chemo, then radiation and finally a hysterectomy.

Through it all, we will remember Kelly's honesty and courage. I would like to recount one night especially that occurred two weeks after her knowledge of the breast cancer. One evening, Kelly had gone to her church to light a candle and say some prayers. Church doors locked tight, she crawled into the back seat of her car, rolled into a ball and began to sob in disbelief. Soon the phone rang and I answered to a small childlike voice, crying, "Mom, I'm in the church parking lot. I'm scared; can you pray with me?" I listened quietly while she poured out her fears. I could picture her lying there in the back seat.

Then, as we prayed together, she was able to go home with peace and a feeling of calm. I tried to put myself in her place that night and remember thinking, "My daughter's a remarkable woman." She had very few moments of despair again.

Another occasion, when Kelly was home with her family for a visit, she decided to take a nap on our loveseat by the fireplace. We were accustomed to seeing her without her cap or wig, but that evening as we stole close to peek at her sleeping by the fire, her baldhead was a sad reminder to us of her sufferings. I remembered her baldhead at birth, thirty-eight years ago.

Kelly continued to work all through her treatments and surgeries. She even made plans to return to St. Cloud State University to begin her Master's program. Today, her dream, to become a school counselor is a reality. She is in the midst of her classes and relishes every busy minute of her life, and Kelly has armloads of compassion to give. Since her fight with cancer, she chose to direct her efforts to bring healing to children at risk with her decision to become a school counselor.

It's been nearly three years since that bright carefree day in July, the day all of our lives changed dramatically. Kelly is busy; busy living her life with joy. She experienced the three-day sixty-mile walk for cancer with two dear friends. She is in the middle of her Master's program at SCSU, maintaining an 'A' average and working besides. Kelly speaks at cancer rallies and healing retreats.

She shares that Faith, Family and Friends carried her through those difficult times. Her hair is nearly shoulder length, another triumph. She receives bi-yearly check-ups, and is a survivor of breast cancer: A SURVIVOR! Cancer changed all of our lives forever. Michaela has written about her experiences as a daughter of a cancer survivor and her essays have helped to manage her fears.

Every day, I pray and make a conscious effort not to worry about Kelly's future. I am amazed at her calmness and trust. She simply replies, "I'm looking forward, not backward. Life is an adventure to be lived joyfully each day." And, I couldn't agree more.

A COWGIRL WITH A WILL TO SURVIVE

Sharyl Saver

August 9, 2010

My story with canser* begins one spring morning in April of 2007. While getting ready for work, my youngest son, Jacob, came into my room to give me a hug. He gently put his head on my chest, and I felt something tender. After enjoying his sweet hug, I touched the tender spot and felt a lump. Fear and panic set in.

I felt that lump over and over again for the next couple of days and made an appointment to have it checked out. My doctor decided that it warranted a mammogram, especially considering my family history. My maternal aunt, my mom and five of my maternal great grandmother's sisters all had breast canser. On Tuesday of the following week, I received the news that I had breast canser. I was shocked, devastated and frightened.

How could this be happening to me? My life was going great. I was 36 years old, happily married with three great children, a good job, awesome family and friends. My oldest son was about to graduate from high school. I had two small children and a life to live. I didn't have time for canser. But really, who has time for canser? So, we made decisions.

I went in for a bilateral mastectomy on May 7, 2007. When I woke up from surgery, the first words out of my mouth were "Did it spread to my lymph nodes?" The nurse had to tell me "No" three times before I believed what she said. Even though I was in a lot of pain, I felt an amazing sense of joy. It was the kind of joy you experience when you hold your newborn baby in your arms for the very first time.

As I was transported to my recovery room, I was greeted by my family. I saw smiles on the faces of my husband, my father-in-law, my mom and my dad. I will never forget the joy in my dad's eyes. It is something I go back to often when I am feeling scared or defeated. Although the tumor was small, only 1 cm, and canser had not spread to my lymph nodes, it was a fast-growing canser, and it was recommended that I do four rounds of chemotherapy.

While I was receiving chemo in the summer of 2007, my doctor tested me to see if I was a BRCA carrier based on my family history with breast canser. The BRCA genetic mutations have been proven to increase a woman's lifetime risk of breast and ovarian canser. Not a huge shocker to me when the results came back that I am a carrier. So, in addition to the breast canser blood screenings, my doctor began doing blood tests to screen for ovarian canser.

After I completed chemotherapy in September 2007, I thought I would be able to put this canser stuff behind me and carry on with my life. I began my breast reconstruction process in January of 2008 and completed it in July of that year. My hair was starting to have a style again, and my body was getting back to normal.

Just as things were starting to getting back on track, on October 20, 2008, I received a call from my doctor's office telling me my ovarian tumor marker test was elevated, and she wanted me to do a PET scan. I spent the next six months going through many tests, and in May of 2009, I was diagnosed with a recurrence of breast canser that had metastasized to my liver and two lymph nodes under my left arm. For the last year, I have been doing chemotherapy treatments to eradicate canser from my body.

After my recurrence diagnosis, I received a great book from a group of my friends entitled *Crazy Sexy Cancer Tips* by canser survivor Kris Carr. It"s full of great insights from Kris and her "Cancer Posse," and at the end of the book Kris told me that I was now a "Cancer Cowgirl." (I would be okay with dropping the canser part and just calling myself a cowgirl.)

I have always wanted to be able to call myself a cowgirl. Cowgirls are a tough breed. They may fall but they always saddle up, hold their heads high and ride on. I thought you had to live on a ranch and own a horse to call yourself a cowgirl, but I have learned being a cowgirl is not about where you live; it's a state of mind.

It has been a challenge at times and on occasion my cowgirl spirit has been broken, but I have a great support network that helps restore my cowgirl and faith meters back to full.

My everyday life is filled with more joy than sadness, more hope than disappointment and more love than loneliness. I have awesome friends who encourage me and make me laugh. My parents, brother, sisters and in-laws love me unconditionally, even when I have taken my fears and frustrations out on them. My children love me just because I am their mommy. And, I have my dear, sweet husband and best friend who always stands by my side, constantly cheers me on, never lets me give up, loves me every day, and still looks at me the same way as the day we married. He is my rock and my strength. So, all in all, I would say I am abundantly blessed.

Over the last year, my faith has strengthened deeply. I am not sure how you could get through a bump in the road like this without faith and hope. As a result, I have been so much more aware of the rainbows in my life. Rainbows to me are like a promise of faith and hope that although we may experience rain in our lives some of the most spectacular beauty is created as a result of the rain. And in the words of my favorite little cowgirl, Dolly Parton, "If you want the rainbow, you gotta put up with the rain!"

At the end of the book, *Crazy Sexy Cancer Tips,* Kris Carr says that, "being a canser cowgirl or cowboy is being a part of a divine order, a free-spirited bunch of powerful people who take charge as we gallop through life's obstacle course. We don"t whisper, we ROAR! We are heavenly creatures full of sass and fireworks. We are dazzling warriors full of peace and fury."

I strive every day to live up to this description. Some days, I fall short and others I live up to it beyond my expectations. But mostly, I am proudly just a cowgirl with a will to survive.

Note: Saver intentionally misspelled the word "cancer" to negate its power.

THE NORTH SHORE

Steve Linstrom

The waters of Lake Superior crashed against the dark rock shelf surrounding Isle Royale jubilantly throwing streams of glittering white water diamonds into the air.

From our vantage point on top of the little rise across the bay, we watched our three boys cavorting across the hard crusty surface, dodging the splashes from the incoming surf and stomping in the sparkling little pockets of water. They looked like they were bounding across the face of the moon.

"Terribly brutal, the way the lake relentlessly pounds the island," Molly said, her rich dark brown eyes open impossibly wide. "Year after year, it takes a little piece with each wave. It's terrible but beautiful."

She turned and looked straight into my face. "And in the end—you know—Superior will win and the island is changed forever."

"But the shore changes a little everyday," I said, my fingers running up her spine. "Not all at once. And there is no winner or loser, only change. That's what makes it so beautiful."

She faced the bay again. "Not too close now!" she yelled, her loud mom-ish voice carrying across the water. "And keep your shoes on!"

I smiled. Our "boys" were 25, 23 and 13 and more than capable of watching out for themselves. A mother's instinct to protect is always there. As they have since adolescence, they pointedly ignored their mother's advice. Support her—yes. Listen to her?—no.

"It's relentless and the end is inevitable," I said as a large streamer crashed against the rocks and slowly faded back into the dark body of water. "In some ways, it reminds me of...."

I felt a small shudder from Molly's back. I closed my eyes and silently lowered my chin to my chest. It was always there at the edge of our consciousness. *Christ*, I thought shaking my head. *Even here it's with us. I've managed to do it again.*

I covered her hand in mine and she put her other hand on top, squeezing tightly. I looked at her beautiful face and saw it was scrunched up into her famously ugly grimace. Molly didn't cry very often, up until a year ago that is, but she cried the way she did everything else. All in, full out.

"I'm sorry," I said. "I didn't mean...."

"Just shut the hell up!" she said as a tear made its way down her cheek. "Don't you know we can't be afraid of the word?"

I put my hand behind her head and drew her to my shoulder, my fingers entwined in the thin wisps of hair the chemo had left us.

"Shhhh," I said as I stroked the back of her head. "It's okay. This island has stood up to Superior for millions of years and we'll stand, too."

"I know we will," she said in a whisper. "It's just that I hate this freaking disease. It's just not fair and there just isn't enough time."

I wanted to tell her that everything would turn out okay.

I wanted to tell her that we had time.

I wanted to tell her that they might find a cure.
I wanted to tell her that it hit each person differently.
I wanted to tell her that some people lived with the Beast for years.

She knew. She knew it all. She'd heard it all before. We both heard it all before.
I—can't—fix—anything.

I pulled her head to my shoulder and felt her tears on my neck.
"I know," I whispered. "And I love you. We all love you."

DENIAL

Micky McGilligan

Now I lay me down to sleep,
and pray the Lord my soul to keep.
If I should die before I wake,
I pray the Lord my soul to take.
God bless Mommy and Daddy and Sister and Brother
and make Daddy well.

That was when my brother and I didn't *have* to do anything in particular, except play we were foxes behind the couch, and come when we were called—to dinner, a bath, bedtime. As far as I remember, my brother was always there. We had a big sister around, but she went to school.

Mommy took care of everybody by doing all kinds of things around the house. We didn't think about what that was all about as long as she was there somewhere. We liked it when she made us really neat toys, like doll clothes or blanket forts and when she read picture books to us before we went to bed every night. When we decided to run away from home, she helped us pack. We got half a block down the alley before deciding we didn't know how to get to Gramma's house.

Daddy went to work most days. Sometimes, we picked a tie for him to wear to work. I liked the shiny red one with an anchor sewn in black thread. If we went to the store with him, we weren't supposed to walk *too* fast. Daddy was slow because of the metal brace on his leg and the wooden cane he leaned on. At night, the last words of our prayers were always, "...and make Daddy well." It was just another thing that Mommy taught us to say. I don't think we worried about anybody really dying before we woke. I mean, what was dying anyway?

Seemed like an ordinary life. We hadn't learned yet that options existed, so weren't at a point where we could exercise a lot of choices or even wish for them. You have to grow into knowing that there is anything missing in your family's life.

Two and three became five and six, nine and ten, twelve and thirteen and school came between my brother and I. Being boy and being girl came between us. We didn't think much about drifting apart. There were plenty of other things to think about. Friends. School. Television! I got a job. He sold pot. I was oblivious to that unfortunately.

As we moved through our teens, Dad got slower despite the hospital stays, but he still went to work. Sister went away to college. Mom took care of everybody. I thought Mom did everything perfectly. How wrong could I be? One day, she overdosed on sleeping pills, and left no note of goodbye or why.

By then, my brother and I had not known each other very well at all for several years. I was away at college and he was a senior in high school. "She died of complications from Emphysema" was the official tale. So life went on with us, denial trailing along. Relationships, careers, children or no children, marriages or not. It wasn't all dark for our family, you see, just because we lost a mother and a wife. Take my word for it. Life is good. It goes on. I assure you we were as happy a family as any.

Later, Dad left us the normal way, via heart attack. Maybe the Multiple Sclerosis shortened his life, but he lived it well enough, as well as any of us do, despite his handicaps. This is the way some stories finish. Though the Mom and the Dad are gone from this story, the children live it still.

JEFF COLLA

Not a soul alive walks through life without trials, tribulations and crosses to bear. It is about living and how we cope and deal with these adversities, which makes us who we are. We choose our own paths and approaches and there are wonderful support structures around us, should we need them. We also strangely get a bit closer to God when dark clouds roll in, and maybe it's His special way to keep us near and dear. But as we choose our paths, we all need to be strong and utilize the pillars of what we've learned in life. For me, my approach has been to adopt the 'tudes' as I like to call them. Three self discovered truths to live by. Attitude, Latitude, and Gratitude are the paradigms and partners in my life. They weave through my ever waking moments and are the foundation of my daily being.

Attitude is the essence of how we need start each day. Getting up on the right side of the bed, as they say. This is something we freely choose and an important part of how our day will go. Taking a positive attitude promotes bodily health and well being and walks us down the path to wellness. Positive energy rubs off on to other people as well, and creates an environment for happiness and healing. It's funny, but if you think you are going to get sick, you usually do. The mind is a powerful force in controlling how the body reacts and responds to events. Positive attitudes and thinking coupled with faith can lead to everlasting hope.

The second 'tude' is latitude, the ability to show tolerance and understanding. This is something we learn as we live, grow and observe the world. As we walk through life, situations arise requiring being human and showing compassion. Not everyone or everything is the same and being different in itself is not necessarily wrong or bad. The world still struggles with racism and biases based upon differences such as skin color, religion or politics. Encompassing some latitude in one's life can go a long way to making the world a better place and each of us a better person.

Finally, there is the inner peace of gratitude. A day should not go by where we don't acknowledge how lucky we are to be alive. Yes, we may have our issues, but there is always something to be thankful for. It's all in our perspective and ability to see the goodness in things. One cannot take anything for granted in life. Ours is a fragile existence and we are only on earth for a short time. Find things to be happy about every day and be grateful for them. Make the most of your life with grace, enduring what you must. Even little things can magnify themselves in importance and when health issues arise, the focus becomes even more magnified. Never lose the perspective that things could be worse and be grateful for what we have and who we are.

Nearly ten years ago, as a 48-year-old man, I discovered that I had stage three prostate cancer. In a sense, it was my "wake up" call and now it would become my dark companion for life. After surgery and radiation, the prognosis was that the aggressive cancer would likely return in 2-3 years. Today, I'm happy to report that I'm cancer free and one of the millions of survivors. But I can't help always looking back over my shoulder and wondering if the darkness will return. The disease is currently incurable but much progress is occurring every day. Most of the credit for my remission goes to the grace of God, but He has imparted some wisdom in me as well. My 'tudes', attitude, latitude and gratitude go a long way to giving me a happy life and the means of dealing with the darkness. Life offers many unknowns and situations that call for balance at times. My approach is to use the 'tudes' like a three-legged stool that stands firm no matter what surfaces in life. On this stool, I can stand, balanced and just a little taller, to face all that life has to offer and keep the dark companion at bay. For, I will always be just a bit taller than he is.

CANCER JOURNALS

Shari Albers

December 3

Ten friends gather for the annual holiday dinner and white elephant gift exchange. After Dorothy arrives a bit late, we sit down to a festive potluck dinner. We pass the chicken and baked potatoes, the salad and pickled beets. As we fill our plates, Dorothy clears her throat and asks for our attention. She clasps her fingers and lays her hands on the table. "I need to tell you something," she says. "I want us to carry on and have a good time, but first I need to get this over with." Very clearly, very directly, she says, "I have cancer."

As my eyes fix on the wrinkled skin of my baked potato, I listen to my friend talk about her hospital visit, many tests, and initial diagnosis. Shock. Bewilderment. Numbness. I slowly look up and scan the dazed looks on the others' faces. I bend forward to meet Dorothy's bright eyes and hopeful smile. Twenty-five years flash—career changes, growing families, retreats, five-year plans . . . We know each other's life stories. We reach to grasp each other's hands.

Everyone asks questions. No, the doctor doesn't know what kind of cancer. More tests next week. We eat dinner and then move to the living room. Along the way, I hug Dorothy close. "I'm here for you," I say. "I knew you would be," she replies. We gather around the coffee table filled with colorfully wrapped gifts. We read silly clues and open hilarious re-gifts. We trade treasures and convulse in laughter, shed some tears, and vow support for our friend. But an uninvited eleventh presence hovers and refuses to leave.

December 8

"It's incurable lung cancer," her voice says. My grip on the phone tightens. Appointed to await Dorothy's call after another round of tests, I take the information to further inform our circle of friends. The doctor offered two options, she says. Practical Dorothy comes up with a third. She'll take the new pill and forego the chemo—lesser side effects—maybe a better quality of life. No phone calls or emails from anyone for three days, please.

I don't cry. I keep to task. I take notes, wish her well, hang up, and then I let out an unnatural, piercing howl. How can one's life turn 180 degrees with one phone call? I had come to terms with her "cancer," but how did simple symptoms turn into a death sentence? Most people have at least a chance at conquering cancer, don't they? Good friends are not supposed to die when we are still reaching for our dreams.

January

Dorothy is here, living and looking quite healthy, but she is forever different. I am different. Darkness hovers, as she and I page through information at the Women's Cancer Resource Center, check the progress of new drugs, and find hopeful stories of cancer survivors who beat the odds. Words that were ordinary now have a shift of meaning. The future doesn't look the same anymore—doesn't feel right. It's not my cancer that's following me around like a shadow. It's her cancer. But her cancer is now my cancer. She is my friend—my support—my cheerleader. And I am hers. Now, I must be her rock.

March

I turn calendar pages, schedule upcoming appointments and social activities, and even that routine has a new edge. Will Dorothy still be here on this date? That date? Shall I cancel my upcoming trip? Will the cancer that we didn't know existed in her body six months ago claim her life in a few months? Weeks? Tomorrow?

April

The cancer drug is working. Dorothy's hair and nails have stopped growing. Good signs. We hope the same can be said about the cancer cells.

May

Dorothy is feeling good. Normal, she says. We celebrate her birthday in a big way, all the while wondering if this is her last. She wonders that, too. I ask her how often she thinks of dying. She says those thoughts are bookends to her day. Every day.

June

We focus on writing and having fun at the cabin. I write children's stories. She writes essays about her life with cancer. This time together is full and rich and brilliant. We read our work to each other and discuss the process and impact. Like always, we write quick essays for fun: "Moments of Magic," "Finding Balance," and "Recovery." Then we each make a one-year plan.

December

Everything is illuminated. This life shift has shoved me off my foundation, but it's not all bad. Words, expressions of feelings, and facts all have edges that weren't there before. Some concepts are brilliantly clear, but others are skewed and raw and oddly highlighted. Dorothy laughs at my revelations, but then says she feels it too.

February

"I'm in a Buddhist monk kind of state today," says Dorothy. "Everything is fine as it is." The day spent at a house on the Mississippi feels so right that we write an essay called "The Perfect Day." Then we put pennies on the railroad tracks and wait for trains to come by and flatten them. We laughed so hard last night. We played Scrabble and wrote essays using all the words we made on the board. It feels good to be full of joy, despite the darkness.

December

Dorothy is letting go of few desires—objects—plans. She's not writing much now. She's slowly giving away some of her treasures—Moroccan jewelry, porcelain dolls, African fabrics, books, lace, pottery—things she collected from her worldly travels. Things she cherished. What will it feel like when she lets go of me?

February

Dorothy and I are on another retreat. She can't get comfortable. She doesn't write.

I surrender into my journal and wonder about my life after Dorothy.

Will I hear her voice in the quiet of the woods? Will I sense her laughter in my head or feel her hand upon my shoulder? I don't want to let go.

July

Started my Seven A.M.—Noon shift with Dorothy. For over a month, twenty friends have been administering 24-hour care for her. I'm feeling melancholy. The two big elms in front of my house were marked for death yesterday. I sit here crying for them. For her. For me.

Soon we'll walk around the house again. One very thin friend, wracked with cancer, will hold onto a tall, sturdy friend. Each of us will put one foot in front of the other, slowly pushing forward, for one more round. Her cancer has become our cancer, and we bear it together.

I hold on to these days. I absorb Dorothy's spirit. I feel her strength and resolve. Despite the looming shadow, she emits brilliance.

MY WALK WITH DEATH

Brenda Hartman

I am not supposed to be alive right now. In 1988, my diagnosis was stage four ovarian cancer. According to statistics at that time, I had a five percent chance of living twenty-four months, and no one lived beyond twenty-four months.

I was a graduate student at the University of Minnesota and I was diagnosed between classes. I was working on two PhD's. I went to have an outpatient procedure, because they thought I had endometriosis. It turns out that I had stage four ovarian cancer! They did not expect me to live. I was hospitalized for chemotherapy treatments, had multiple surgeries and two near-death experiences. I had a "spontaneous remission," or I was a "medical mystery," or "a miracle occurred" (many phrases have been used to describe what happened) and I lived. My oncologist told me that I am alive because of what I did, since what they did to me should have killed me.

For over twenty years, I have pondered why I lived. My life path has brought me to many places I never imagined. I shredded two dissertations and started a third which would explore the allopathic and indigenous forms of healing and how they can work together. Then I shredded that dissertation.

Today I am psychotherapist (MSW, LICSW) in private practice with a specialization in oncology. Working with cancer patients, their families and support teams is a gift to me. We talk honestly about the physical, emotional and spiritual experience of living with a life-threatening disease. I walk next to cancer patients when they are in treatment, between treatments, in remission, and, in many cases, as they walk to their death. These patients have honored me by sharing their leaving processes. They have taught me a great deal about life and death. I have also spoken with and studied other cultural responses to death and dying. There is a broad spectrum of beliefs in this world. As I prepared for my own death, and as I help others' prepare for their deaths, my learning from these situations lead me to believe we all have our own beliefs about life and death.

Death can be difficult to discuss. We all have an emotional response to death. Culturally, there is resistance seemingly rising from a belief that anyone talking about death is asking to die. When I was in treatment, I was so sick and in so much pain I wanted to die. But I did not die, even when I wanted to.

There is also the belief that if we talk about dying we are giving up hope. I disagree. When someone is diagnosed with cancer I believe we are all thinking about death; his, hers, mine, yours, those who have died…. It requires a lot of energy to have thoughts about death, and even more to keep them hidden as if there is something wrong with them. When I meet people, death is one of our first discussion topics.

The English language does not have many words to describe death, the feelings around death, or the spiritual changes that many times take place. Because of this, I have created certain terms and phrases to help us communicate about these topics.

People come to me wanting to know how I healed. I know everything in my life lead up to it. It was much more complicated than doing the one right thing. I did many things. One of the most important things I did was to prepare for my death. I did this twice- when I was first diagnosed, and again when I was actively dying, right before my spontaneous remission. I found that by preparing for my death, I could focus all of my energy on living. When thoughts and fears about my death came up, I had a way to respond and could then return my focus to living.

I am not interested in anyone believing what I believe. My intention in stating my beliefs is to provide a still point for others to push against and discover what they believe and why. I believe we all have separate healing paths and our complete healing occurs when we die physically to this earth. So I suggest, when asking for healing, ask only for a 95% healing so one can stay in the physical world.

Since my second near-death experience, I think/see mentally in pictures. It is as though the door between this world and the other world (where we go when we die) was blown off and I can no longer close the door. Images come through to me. I have used these images or pictures to help me describe concepts when I am meeting with cancer patients. One image of life and death is that we are all walking on the road of life. We each have a personal fork on the road which leads off the main road and takes us to our physical death. To consciously live and consciously die, we become aware of, and look for, our personal fork in the road.

When a cancer patient is first diagnosed, for many people it is their first sense of their own death. Prior to that experience, we all walk around knowing about death, saying, "it happens to all of us," and "you can't get out of here alive," but we don't really have a sense of what that might mean. When cancer patients are with me, we discuss ways to prepare for death/healing while actively living. I refer to this as "coming even with life and death." One of my first homework assignments for my patients is to create a list of things they want to complete before they die. We discuss wills, funeral plans, obituaries, dispersal of physical property, letters to be written, and all the other details of life that an individual may want to complete. This list is different for each person. Following that, we move on to what needs to occur to say goodbye to the people we love. This brings a person into consciously living each moment they have with their loved ones. On multiple occasions, I have witnessed the relief of stress upon completion of this list. Patients focus on living each moment and they live moments/days/weeks/months/years longer than was ever predicted by the medical statistics. I call this game "stump the docs." While scratching their heads, the docs respond with "I don't know why you are doing as well as you are, but we are pleased about it."

I imagine us having two parts—the physical body, which I refer to as a "vessel," and our spirit or soul—that part which leaves the physical body when we say that a person has died. I have witnessed individuals consciously walking to their physical death on their fork in the road and many times they have awareness from both parts of themselves, their physical body/mind and spirit/soul on the other side. Often when people are in both places at once, they are able to speak from both places. Many times I have heard people use the term "we" when they are speaking from their spirit/soul perspective. I understand the use of "we" to refer to words coming from the individual's soul in connection with other souls: Great Spirit, God, Jesus, Allah, Waken Tankan, the One who goes by a Thousand Names and the One who is Nameless. This is difficult to explain in English words. In all cases, when I have heard individuals using the word "we" in this way, there was something which clarified their intention to be speaking from the point of view of a collective, something greater than the individual's personal understanding or knowing.

Many individuals in an active dying state have shared with me a variety of thoughts, including: they can feel/tell that "my door" to the other side is open, that they trust me to guide them to the other side; they know I will walk over with them so they will not be alone, etc. The first time I was told this I was surprised and confused. I wondered what they saw and felt when they were with me. I have been told this many times now, so I am no longer surprised and find comfort in trusting that my soul and the soul of the individual telling me this are working together, beyond my conscious understanding.

My cancer forced me to face my death. It was a "twisted gift," my phrase to represent events that begin so painful but bring healing and beauty into your life.

I believe that preparing for my death; completing things, saying my good byes, completing the paper work I felt necessary, etc., allowed me then to focus all my energy on healing. To this day, I do not know why I lived but I do know that I live a happier life. It is easier to know what is important in *my* life.

WHEN THERE ARE NO MORE WORDS

Kelly Paradis

The silence is what I notice most. My parents still call almost every Sunday evening, each on a handset, both on the line, telling me about their week from different rooms. They have done this since I was in college, when I would call home under the guise of talking about my classes but also hinting and hoping for a few more dollars in my checking account to cover those late night pizza orders. Sometimes, they would bicker on the line, contradicting each other while giving their best advice on how to cook a meatloaf, or whether I should be concerned about a cough that was lingering. When my husband and I moved to Canada, they worried long distance in my ear each week about whether we were working too hard or if it made sense to make the twenty-one hour drive home for Christmas.

Now they are in Arizona for half the year and my mother is in the early stages of Alzheimer's. She is seventy-one and has been diagnosed for two years. She says hello excitedly when we all get on the phone and shares a few things about what they have done that week, but then she is quiet, and I have to remind myself that it's not just Dad on the line. Sometimes, he cues her and asks her specific questions about something that they have done—a trip to the coffee shop, a dinner with friends. She remembers most of it, but I can hear her reaching deep for the words, struggling to find the term that describes what they were doing a few hours ago - sitting outside on the sidewalk, talking to people at the coffee shop, petting the dogs that stroll by with their owners past the benches where they drink their coffee.

"We saw Coach!" she says, happy to remember the name of a regular. "You'd like him," she adds. "I'll introduce you when you come down to visit. He's a very nice man." I don't mention to her that I have met Coach many times over the last eight years that they have been spending the winter down south.

"He used to work in the high school here," she says. "I think he taught something."

"He was a basketball coach," my dad adds, reminding my mom that this is how he got the name.

"Oh, that's right" she says thoughtfully and is quiet again.

"That makes sense," I say. "I'll look forward to meeting him. I'll bet he's very nice."

My dad continues talking, telling me about the concert they just saw, the dinner with neighbors, their recent phone call with my sister and her kids and of course, the weather. The weather is a big part of our conversation. My parents love to hear about the snow they are missing and the sub-zero temperatures. Mom tells me about the hummingbird they saw out the window and I ask her if she has been sitting outside on the porch enjoying the sunshine. She tells me that they watched a funny show last night, but as she starts to describe it, she forgets what it is called. She gives me enough description for me to guess "Ally McBeal."

"That's it!" she says excitedly. "It's so funny."

Dad tells me about two of their neighbors who are having a dispute over not raking pine needles in a timely manner. He mentions that he has talked to both of them and they are each pointing the finger at the other person and neither one wants to rake them up.

"Who are we talking about again?" my mom asks.

"Tom and Nancy," my dad says, "they can't agree on who has to rake."

"Oh?" says Mom, "Do they live by you, Kelly?"

"No, Tom and Nancy—the people on the corner here," my dad says, sounding slightly annoyed that Mom is not tracking the conversation.

"Oh, yeah, Tom and Nancy," she repeats back and is quiet again for a long stretch.

My mother has her master's degree in education and has spent a lifetime teaching children to read their first words. She covered my bedroom in construction paper letters and taught me the alphabet before I was three. She read me books every day and each night before bed. I started Kindergarten being able to read, write and spell.

I have my mother and her mother to thank for my love of reading and writing. It runs in our family. My maternal grandmother also had her master's degree in education and taught school until my mom was born. She was part of a contesting club, writing original advertising slogans and jingles for contests in the 1950s. She won cars, washing machines, appliances and vacations and kept a scrapbook full of her entries. This was back when they awarded prizes for originality and not just random drawings. Grandma adored Victorian literature and made up elaborate bedtime stories for us based on her favorite books, putting my sister and me in as characters in some of the tales.

My grandma had a stroke in her late seventies and began to have a hard time remembering the right words. I would watch her struggle to find the name for the white thing that she wanted to cut up and put in the salad.

"Iron?" she would say, looking in the cupboards. "You know, round, makes you cry."

"Onion," I'd say, and she would nod and sigh, disappointed that her brain was letting her down. She developed macular degeneration, a reverse tunnel vision where she could only read on the outside periphery of her vision. She gave up her daily Scramble puzzles and crosswords and reading the newspaper. Dementia crept in and it became harder to hold a conversation with her without it devolving into stories of neighbors stealing precious books and antiques from her home. Of all the things she lost during her last years, losing her ability to read was the hardest to take.

My mother is still reading. She got a Nook for Christmas and with my dad's help has downloaded *Little Women* onto it. I ask her on the phone if she's still reading it.

"Page 187," she says proudly, "Jo has just cut off her hair."

"I remember that part," I say. "I should read those books again. I always loved Louisa May Alcott."

"I don't think I've ever read her before," my mom says and I cheerfully encourage her to check out "Little Men" when she finishes this one.

"I will," she says. "I'll bet it's good."

"It is," I say. "I think you'll like them."

I look over at my bookshelf. The leather-bound copy of *Little Women* sits next to *Jo's Boys* and *Little Men*—books from my mother's well-read childhood. She is discovering them again, for the first time in her mind, and it is making her happy. I am glad that books still give her joy and whether she remembers the words tomorrow or next month, she is happy today and that is what matters.

EVERY LITTLE THING

Nathan R. Miller

He sat as upright as his weakening muscles would allow while closing his eyes and turning his face upward to the penetrating Caribbean sun. He may have raised his arms, palms outstretched, but it would have been fleeting. The strength simply was not there. The four of them bobbed on their little catamaran in the bay as the rest of us fought back tears that were dropping into the sand massaging our bare feet.

Don't worry about a thing, 'cause every little thing gonna be all right.

My sister mentioned during a series of email exchanges one January that her husband was going in to the doctor to ask about some trouble he had been experiencing while trying to speak and swallow food. He also had a muscle twitch that just wouldn't stop, even keeping him up at night. She didn't come across as too concerned until the doctor referred him to a specialist for testing, with a note for the specialist that read "Neurodegenerative disorder?" Times such as they are, patients oftentimes turn to the Internet for instant medical knowledge, and searches for neurodegenerative disorders brought up all kinds of information on diseases like MS. Further studying of well-intentioned (but anxiety-producing) online lists of symptoms suggested that a more likely match was in fact ALS, or Lou Gehrig's disease.

When the diagnosis came back confirming the worst, I frantically searched for information anywhere I could get it. The more I read, the more it seemed this disease was some insidious form of torture in the worst possible order. Patients with ALS literally wither. Of sound mind but not body, connections between the brain and the muscles die off, leaving patients weak, dependent, immobile, and eventually unable to eat and breathe.

It is a death sentence, with no explanation, reason, or recourse. Cause and cure both elude researchers, and the average life expectancy of two to five years after diagnosis does not provide much of a window for any medical advancements to be of use to current patients. To hear ALS explained is to hear the sound of abstract helplessness expressed in word form, yet the rallying cries of people affected by ALS everywhere continue to be words and phrases like *hope* and *never give up*. Obviously, John's diagnosis was a devastating blow to his immediate family and all of his surrounding loved ones.

So when, not even a month after the diagnosis, the call came to say John wanted to take a vacation and he hoped as many people would join him as possible, there was no doubt my wife and I would go along. We had turned down plenty of getaway invitations in the past, but there was no missing this one. In a matter of just a few weeks, rooms were booked, tickets were purchased, and twelve siblings, in-laws, and friends were Jamaica-bound to celebrate our connection to a good man facing unimaginable prospects.

Such a trip would have been exciting regardless, but what we all kept thinking about—while looking at Caribbean Sea photos online during February in Minnesota—was just how much we all needed something positive to focus on. I know that there was no stopping

Stephanie and John from dwelling on the impending ramifications of his disease, but at least there was now something else to think about.

I remember clearly now, looking back, how walking behind John at the airport on the way to our departure gate was the first time his deterioration was visibly obvious to me. He had a rigidness to his step that at times was quite subtle, and at others it seemed to nearly trip him. It was as if the traction on the bottoms of his shoes was too strong; there was no fluidity to his walk. The casual observer most likely would have completely overlooked his stinted gait, but in the weeks following John's formal diagnosis we all fell into a trap of unintentionally scanning his every word and motion for signs of symptoms progressing.

Don't worry about a thing, 'cause every little thing gonna be all right.

For one week, we got to help Stephanie and John live in carefree luxury. We had collectively and secretly upgraded their room to a massive suite, complete with two-tiered balcony and outdoor spa tub. Red Stripe, Appleton, and rum cream concoctions flowed freely from the pool bars, not even requiring us to get out of the water and face the demands of such inconveniences as having to bear our full weight while walking. Reggae music played from every direction, as if Bob Marley himself simply hung in the air unobtrusively, turning the gentle rustle of the breeze into repetitions of "no worries."

In fact, Marley's tribute to his back-up singers (his wife among them—even more appropriate given the enormous challenges facing John's wife as his primary caregiver), turned into our mantra during our stay. Every time we heard *Three Little Birds,* we were swept up in a mindset of casting all our fears, including omnipresent Death, aside. ALS is so damning in its certainty, its unflinching mortality, that it's difficult to think about anything other than what you know is coming—and coming with horrific speed. Yet the magic of everything aligning allowed us all, John and Stephanie included, to forget it all for just a moment and to truly feel no worries. Close friends and family united in an idyllic setting where celebrating life was part of the very culture...it was just the right medicine at just the right time.

In the years since, I have found the song evokes sweet nostalgia and bitter resentment. At times, it's almost as if the words mocked me: there was plenty to worry about; it was not all going to be all right. Above all else, however, I am grateful.

We all face the same mortality John faced, but most of us get to live with a certain amount of denial. At the very least, our eventual deaths are not realities we need to dwell on regularly. Before he even had a chance to turn forty, John found out he likely had two to five years left of his life. The lust for life he displayed each remaining day, coupled with his wife's heroic efforts to bear the burden of his increasing needs on top of all other obligations, served as inspiration to us all. Memories of John—before, during, and following Jamaica—reminded us all that it would be best to try and treat more days, more gatherings, and more time as celebrations of life and those who make it livable.

Don't worry about a thing, 'cause every little thing gonna be all right.

At face value, the idea behind the lyrics is so silly, so sentimentally optimistic... but it still provides me with the warming comfort of a tropical noonday sun. I close my eyes, imagine John out on the water, and know that it is possible for a second, a minute, or even a whole week for everything to be all right.

SOLACE

Deborah Gordon Cooper

My Father

Wears his slippers
to my brother's house
for Sunday brunch.
His old, gray mukluks
pace the yard
and clutch at twigs
and leaves and bugs.

I watch his feet,
and then I watch
the bright wool
of his heavy sweater
move across the grass,
again and back,
in the hot May sun.

Close-up is always hardest.
His eyes, behind smudged glasses,
seem now smudged themselves
and far away.
I want to clean them off
so he can really look
at me again.

I wipe his chin,
make it a joke
to save him from disgrace.
Perhaps he is beyond
embarrassment.
I hope so, but then right away
I hope not yet.

We drive home in the dark
in the thick, sad silence
that always comes after.
I imagine my real father

in his wing-tips, perfect shirt
and tie, waiting somewhere
for the rest of him to come.

From the back seat
my son's hand
finds my shoulder
and I remember telling him
once years ago
that there was no such thing
as purgatory.

The Letter

My father, who can't remember
what he had for lunch
or if he's eaten anything at all,
tells me that once
trying to win my mother's heart
he had made a letter
out of flower petals
and sent it to her in the mail.
He must've been nineteen.
And I imagine him, unfastening
the daisies from their orbs,
undoing blue-bells and
reorganizing asters.

My mother remembers then too.
Remembering makes her face go soft
and shine right on him
in a way I have not seen in years.
And I can see her, opening
the envelope that day,
the same look softening her face
as if a breeze had crossed it.
Somewhere, out of sight,
a gate swings open.

Practicing

My father only wants to eat
Eskimo-pies.

I bring a new box every Sunday.
He leaves them, melting
and forgotten, on the couch,
between the pages of the books
he cannot read but carries everywhere,
as if they hold his old identity.
My father can no longer tie his shoes.
He waits for me to,
sitting meekly in the chair.
I remember sitting on the stairs
of the old house
while he taught me how,
before kindergarten, on the day
of the shoe scramble.
I swallowed my crying then too,
afraid that it would be too hard.
I tie carefully, the way he
taught me, making the laces
even, using double-knots.
He is talking, something about the sky
outside the window
and the war,
loses hold of the thought,
dozes off between words.
I look up at him, his face
collapsed against his chest, traces
of chocolate on his chin, slipping out
of the world, as if he is
practicing leaving it.

Reasons

Because there is so little
left blooming,
each delinquent petal
seems to shine.

Because the sun is pulled
behind the hills
a little earlier each day,
I wake in time
to catch it rising.
Because my father

is forgetting
how to talk,
I make a treasure
out of every
awkward utterance.

The Benevolent Doorman

Because, growing up,
I'd heard you say,

"Pneumonia is the old man's friend."

I recognized him
when he came for you.

Visitations

On Tuesday, in the produce aisle,
choosing my oranges by feel
and by their fragrance,
I hear my father whistling in my ear.
A Scottish lullaby.
Everything else stops.

There is a tenderness no border can contain.
A web that may be glimpsed
in certain, unexpected plays of light,
or felt, like a shawl
across one's shoulders,
laid by unseen hands.

There are sounds in other decibels
the heart can hear, when the wind is right
and the mind has quieted its clicking.
The border guards are sleeping
at their stations.
Spirits come and go.

The wall between the living and the dead
is as yielding as a membrane,
is as porous as a skin.

Lay your palm against it
and you can hear their voices in your hand
and in the place where the chest opens
like a flower.

They are not far away,
no farther than the breath
and enter us as easily,
in pine and peonies
in oranges and rain.

Solace

And still
the world goes on
being beautiful...
the trees, the water and the sky
offering solace,
whether we see or not.

Just now, the clouds
behind the black limbs
of the mountain ash
catch fire in the last light
of the day.

Hope rings
in the delicate throat
of a single bird,
singing the sun down,
whether we're listening
or not.

Even as we sleep
the gracious moon
traces the sky
keeping the night-watch,
soft spill of light
across the bed.

LYNN J. MCLEAN

Hearing yet again the advantages of my tongue cancer being caught early while still small may cause me to scream. This is the third time. Other cancers, older and larger, have responded to treatment. After one surgery and thirty-five sessions of radiation, mine hasn't. "Radiation Failure," they said. Even now, the words make me nauseous. Radiation is hell and left lasting damage, except to my cancer.

Two years ago, on my first visit with the oral surgeon, the worst case scenario he'd outlined was where I am now in the place no one believed I'd be. After all, my cancer had been caught early and was small. The first biopsy indicated "precancerous."

After my first surgery, which lasted four hours longer than expected, the surgeon said it looked like "slow-growing" cancer. Two weeks later, the report said, "aggressive." At warp speed, I went from optimistic to cautiously optimistic to struggling to be optimistic. But still it was early and small....

In no way do I match the profile for oral cancer. Statistically, this should not have happened. I conclude that statistics have their place, I guess. But what matters is what's happening to me. Despite favorable odds, I've eluded them all.

For me, "arrival" is misleading. It suggests a single event. I wish. My cancer arrives again and again. It arrives in successive diagnoses, in ongoing losses, and in changing relationships. The earth under me unendingly shifts and slides. Only it's not under me; it's inside of me. It is me. It is my body.

My six adult children appeared to ignore my diagnosis, even after the first surgery that removed a small portion of my tongue. To them it was a minor "fender bender." After some tweaking, I was as good as new. Statistically they were right.

But I'd had friends who died of cancer. There is no "fender bender" cancer. I knew I could die. Death weighed heavily. Eventually, I realized "It's not about death; it's about living." Naively, I believed my cancer was gone. Instead, it was on hiatus and reappeared thirteen months later.

All three times, I found my cancer first as a sore on my tongue that hurt badly. My body knew; my mind rejected. So, while my intellect was crushed each time, my core remained unsurprised when cancer was confirmed, confirmed, confirmed.

The second time, doctors recommended radiation. Going nearly daily thirty-five times felt like going to my execution, though sessions were non-events. You start out feeling not so good and gradually it got worse, with the end the worst. I thought I'd die. Without concerted caring by family and friends, I think I might have. The kindnesses from those known and unknown made all the difference during every phase.

Some weeks after radiation, I had a nightmare. I woke mumbling, "Oh, no, Oh, no, Oh, no." Even awake, the dread did not pass. It sank into my soul. Then a sore surfaced in my mouth where the cancer had been. No one wanted to believe it was cancer again. But it was.

The biopsy was done at the beginning of the week. I was leaving to visit friends at the end of the week. My husband was out of the country. I made the surgeon promise to call and tell me the outcome. By early Friday afternoon, as I still hadn't heard, I called and spoke with a resident. Residents haven't honed the persona of their teachers. He stammered out one explanation after another. Finally, he said the surgeon would call me. It didn't take a psychic to know things didn't look good. The surgeon called and gave me the bad news—Radiation Failure. He kept saying how sorry he was to have to tell me this. And I know he was. At last I blurted out, "You have to tell me; it's your job."

I had a brief conversation with the radiologist. She told me what a terrible weekend she'd had. She went on to say she'd double-checked everything, and there were no mistakes. Her message was how badly she felt but I never got past her bad weekend. "Lady," I wanted to say, "I'm having a bad life."

The first words I heard were the words that stuck. *Radiation failure.* My ability to comprehend was compromised. Having someone with me when interacting with doctors was crucial. I needed someone to hear and remember and help me "get it." I learned that doctors get very little training in delivering bad news, and the more the doctor cares, the harder it is. My doctors cared a lot.

The surgery I had hoped to avoid with radiation seemed desirable now. This was the last ditch scenario made even "ditchier" by the damage to my tissue from radiation. Forty percent of my tongue plus lymph nodes would be removed. A hunk of flesh and an artery from my forearm would constitute my new tongue. I would have a tracheotomy. Recovery would take a year. Speaking and swallowing would be difficult. My surgeon called it "life altering." Those words were a drop of water in what would be a tsunami in my life.

I almost did not have it done. I'd followed medical recommendations. The cancer was still going strong. There had been traumas in my life that made this surgery seem nearly impossible. I decided that, unless something inside me provided a clear message to go ahead, I would not. I was at a point of exhaustion and grief that made dying acceptable.

Transformation is like "arrival." It is not a single event. I sought out people wise in orthodox and unorthodox ways. I needed to bring meaning to this devastation. In my search, transformation was incremental. Slowly, new insights replaced old beliefs. Peace increased and fear was released.

I had the surgery and confounded everyone with my phenomenal recovery (which felt less than phenomenal to me). My new tongue "took" with no complications. Speaking and swallowing came early. Yet, my speaking is greatly altered. Swallowing does not equal eating. Mostly I drink Ensure and that's not likely to change. Daily, I do exercises for my neck, swallowing, edema, hand, voice, facial paralysis, and shoulder. Yes, shoulder! I have a twenty percent chance of living five years. Love those statistics....

That food is at the core of socializing hits hard. While others read menus and compare entrees, I fiddle with a fork I will not use. As they eat, I drink Ensure. Sometimes I think of myself as a different species that eats and lives differently. One species does not wish to be another. Reframing helps make what seems unbearable possible. I often say to my husband when I don't want to do something, "My species doesn't do that."

Sometimes, I cry for what was. Sometimes, I factor a shortened life expectancy into purchases. If I buy the expensive refrigerator, I may not get my money's worth. Yet, I know more deeply than most that now is the time to do, say, and live what is important. *Later* may not exist, for me or for any of us. This is knowing—hard earned.

KATHERINE MORROW

My illness, breast cancer, has been sitting inside of my breast for a few years now. I haven't wanted to do anything about it because the treatments seemed worse than having a few harmless lumps in my breast. Now I know that those lumps were not as harmless as they seemed.

This fall, when my husband and I were on a trip to Italy, I found out how much damage a little cancer can do. I had a sore leg from yoga before we left for our trip, but the stress of the trip, plus the fact of being caught in a flash flood exacerbated the injury. While walking to dinner in Florence, my leg gave out completely. I cried out in agony as people stared. I couldn't go on. We had a bite to eat at the little outdoor cafe where I had slumped in a chair, but I could just barely walk back to our hotel that was only half a block away. My husband had to carry me up the last ten steps of a long flight of stairs to our room. I was in such pain that I could not sleep and we wondered what we should do. We had reserved a rental car for the next few days and we reasoned that with a few days of rest in the country, my leg would be better.

Jim carried me to the taxi that took us to our rental car, and with the help of a GPS we found our way to Castellina in Chianti where we had reserved a hotel room. The room was beautiful in the classic Tuscan style, but I saw little of the grounds and less of the quaint little village. The only way I got anywhere over the next few days was if my husband carried me. I was getting more and more exhausted because I could not get comfortable enough to sleep. The kind clerks as the Hotel Salviopoli offered to call us a doctor and we finally took them up on it.

The doctor made a house call to our room. After a brief examination, he pantomimed a fist drooping in his palm indicating a broken hip. Without hesitation, he called an ambulance and in another half an hour we were on our way to Siena—the nearest large town with a hospital. I waited for an hour in an emergency room to talk to a doctor about my condition. In broken English, I was questioned about my medications and medical conditions as I lay on a gurney. An X-ray was ordered and I was wheeled down the hall for that. After being wheeled back to the emergency room, my husband was finally able to see me. I was further questioned and finally admitted that I had a lump on my breast. The X-ray must have revealed something concerning because I was then wheeled to the orthopedic wing of the hospital.

More doctors arrived to talk to my husband and me about my prognosis. It appeared that my leg was broken. The petite Dr. Maria Antoinetta Liberati printed off a copy of a thigh bone and then drew a big line across the top to illustrate to my husband the problem. The head doctor—a tiny man wearing orange pants under his white coat with fancy eye glasses —told my husband that they would have to rebuild the bone and that it could be done in a week or so. The cancer doctors were also called in and I was to have a mastectomy and chemotherapy. It was really more than my husband and I could take in.

Although I stayed in the hospital for three more days, my husband and I finally decided that we couldn't have such serious medical treatments in a place where we did not know the language. Dr. Liberati helped us to get an ambulance ride to Pisa where we caught our plane. My husband had to carry me on the plane, but we were able to get wheelchair help through the airports.

After returning, my husband and I were referred to the St. Cloud Hospital by our local physician. The next day I was in the St. Cloud Hospital—a much nicer facility than the one in Siena—and a few days after that I had surgery. I had a total hip replacement. The doctor reported that there was a large tumor in my femur that had broken the leg.

It's been two months now and I am getting treatment for both my breast and bone cancer. I am limping around—still healing from hip replacement. I don't think I ever would have done a thing about the breast cancer if I hadn't broken my leg. I do regret this and I hope that I can serve as an example of what not to do. Cancer doesn't go away. It metastasizes. If I would have treated this a few years ago, I wouldn't have bone cancer. I might have had a mastectomy, but I would be over with this cancer now and able to go on with my life. A friend my mine told me that her mother had a mastectomy fifty years ago and she is alive today. My physical therapist said that her mother had breast cancer forty years ago. The cancer has returned—but forty years is a long time. I hope that I can leave my cancer behind in a year or so, but the statistics are not on my side. All I can do now is take care of myself and have a positive attitude, but I wish it wouldn't have taken a physical breakdown for me to get wise to the damage cancer can do.

THIRTY-EIGHT DAYS

Beret Griffith

My husband Ron and I are at the cabin for the summer.

It's June twenty-second and we're moving heavy fence sections into the woods. You are noticeably tired. By evening, you are dizzy, nauseated and do not eat supper.

After a restless night, breakfast goes untouched; you have indigestion. Alarmed, I wonder "heart attack"? We leave immediately for the Urgent Care Clinic forty miles away. An EKG indicates no heart attack, a relief. Since your blood count is high, you're anemic and have blood in your stool you're being sent to the hospital emergency room. I get the car to pick you up. At the door, nurse runs out saying "Your husband has passed out, was given an IV and an ambulance will take him." I drive myself to Luther hospital.

A gastroenterologist will do a low risk procedure in the morning. You're given blood, are resting and it's a relief to see you under white sheets—blood dripping into your veins. I drive back to the lake.

The procedure takes ten minutes. The camera in your stomach shows three small ulcers. Your hemoglobin, dangerously low, requires you receive more blood. Healing should be complete in ten weeks. I drive myself back to the cabin. The next day, you are released from the hospital, feeling better, ulcer medication and treatment plan in hand. You will see your doctor in a few days. We're looking forward to spending time at the cabin.

June twenty-forth, we drive home. On the way, you make a doctor's appointment for July third.

During the night, your tongue begins to swell. You take an Allegra. The swelling increases. You get up and take another Allegra. I look closely at you, tongue so swollen you can barely mumble a few words, struggling to breathe. I take off pajamas, put on some clothes, order you into the car and say, "We're not going to wait at home to see how this turns out." The emergency room nurse checks your oxygen. You are breathing with difficulty. "Are you going to give Ron an epinephrine shot?" I ask. "I can't" she says, "The doctor has to give it." You can't swallow your saliva and have a towel in front of your mouth. I say, "Where is the ER doctor?" I'm assured he is being located. You're breathing through your nose. The doctor arrives, gives you a shot of Benadryl; the nurse draws blood and you pass out! You're admitted to the hospital for observation, then armed with an epi pen, are sent home. You are itching.

On Monday, June thirtieth, our son calls to tell us his wife just had their fourth healthy daughter. We take care of their other three girls for a couple of days, then drive to the cabin.

On July fifth, you are irritable, off Allegra, itching like crazy and taking meds for swelling. You are not feeling well and nap in the hammock.

Starting today, July nine, we'll have two granddaughters at the cabin for a week. We're excited and anticipate a less eventful week in the health department. We have a wonderful week with the girls. Your itching continues.

On July sixteenth, we drive our granddaughters home. Over the next week, you itch more and more and medication isn't helping. On July twenty-third, at home talking with our daughter-in-law, a nurse, she says, "Have you had a liver enzyme test? "No." On July twenty-fifth, you have the test in the morning and we return to the lake.

At the cabin, several messages from your doctor are on the cabin phone. "Your liver functions are extremely high. Call me right away." You call. He says, "The hospital should have called you with results earlier; go to the hospital as soon as possible." We leave for the emergency room. You're checked in immediately and given a CT scan that reveals enlarged liver ducts. Because it's the weekend, you're released from the hospital and told to come back Monday for a pre-op appointment for an ERCP (Endoscopic Retrograde Cholangiopancreatography) to be done on Tuesday.

We have Saturday and Sunday to mull over what's happening. At the cabin, you go to bed. I Google "ERCP" and find it's done when pancreatic ducts are suspected to be narrowed or blocked due to a possible infection or cancer.

Saturday, we go to our favorite state park. You have only enough energy to rest on a blanket. We lie there, saying little. Our extended family is now aware of what has been happening.

I put a poem by Teresa of Avila in my journal.

Sunday, July twenty-seven, is beautiful. We are keeping negative images at bay. We talk though you have no energy and sleep most of the day.

Monday, July twenty-eighth is the pre-op appointment. You've lost fourteen pounds. A young doctor explains the Tuesday test. The weight of the past month is taking a toll on us. We're tired. Tomorrow will give us a clearer sense of the situation. We feel the potential life-changing quality of the next hours and the need to be ready for whatever comes. So much has happened since moving fence pieces in June and especially since getting the liver enzyme test. We drive back to the lake. As we climb into bed, windows open, hearing comforting night sounds, we talk. I am tearful and you say, "I'm more worried about you than I am about myself."

July twenty-ninth we drive to the hospital. It's a hot, muggy day. I haven't slept much.

You're prepped for the ERCP. The doctor comes in, looks at your CT scan and says, "Well, let's take a look at the tumor." This is the first we've heard the word "tumor." The doctor is surprised and irritated we're not aware of the tumor and have not seen the CT scan. We were to have seen and discussed it at the pre-op appointment. Tears come, yet there is no time for conversation before you're wheeled off.

A pager will notify me when you're in recovery. Now I wait. I'm fearful of calling the kids and tell myself "Take it in, stay open. Receive don't resist." It helps. But I am afraid.

The minutes tick by. Whatever happens may change life as we know it. A small camera is wending its way to your pancreas, liver, gall bladder to look at what has been invading your body without your knowledge or consent. Like a Swiss Army knife on a camera, it can diagnose, sometimes fix, and reveal work of an unseen force.

You're wheeled into the recovery room at 2:15 P.M. The nurse says, "A stent was put into your intestine. The doctor will come in about an hour." I make calls to family and friends. You're groggy and ask whom I've called. I give you water and you sleep.

3:30 PM—you're drowsy, still no doctor. You gradually awaken. After a four-hour wait, the doctor comes in to deliver the diagnosis. "Lymph nodes tested positive for cancer. You have poorly-differentiated, metastatic, Stage IV Pancreatic Cancer. I've made an appointment for you at Mayo to discuss treatment." Short and clear. He continues, "Most people don't live beyond three to six months. You may live longer because you're in otherwise good health." Using the term "good health" in this situation strikes me as odd. As the emotional impact of the news begins sinking in, hand-in-hand we talk about living life fully.

I write DAY ONE in my journal.

NANCY MARATTA

Under the celestial sphere of a starkly cold, silent and unforgiving Alaska winter, my life's journey of fifty-five years—years of good health, boundless opportunities, and the recent immersion into the Yu'pik Eskimo culture—seemed to be at its apex.

Weathered in with five other *bush* teachers, two dogs and my cat, Bearpaw, I was snuggling down into my arctic parka when the call came. As my companions boarded planes to their villages, I headed back to Anchorage on the Big Bird, an affectionate term for the prop planes that flew between Bethel and Anchorage, summoned by a call from my husband, Gene. Evidently, my recent mammogram had raised a few alarms.

My reaction that first evening was simply one of frustration. As the only special education teacher in Tuntutuliak, I took a mental inventory of which children were scheduled for meetings and interventions, surmising that a few days away from the village would not be the end of the world.

What I could not know was that I would never again enter my school building to be greeted by the most beautiful children on this earth, I would never hear the sweet, soft, guttural sound of Yup'ik voices enveloping me or feel my aide's arm around me as we worked out a challenging program for a child. I would never again see and experience the sheer beauty of the Alaskan Bush. The trust and respect from my Yup'ik colleagues and friends that was in its incipience after a short four months in their village—would any of it have had meaning? What would happen to the complex educational plans that would need to be implemented for the children?

It was January 18th 2000, that I arrived back in Eagle River, where my husband kept the home fires burning, and flew back and forth to be with me. After five harrowing days of diagnostic tests, and a visit to the surgeon, my body was lifted up and down onto the cold metal slabs, injected, poked, subjected to sentinel node mapping, a lumpectomy and an axillary dissection. Ah, but that was the easy part. When my pathology report confirmed 3 positive lymph nodes, the stakes got higher; I went from the surgeon to the oncologist and right into treatment.

It was then that the fragile mind—body connection, the usually "together" *Nancy-moving-forward-in-the-world,* started to shift. I became intensely self-reflective. To choose a treatment option, I would need to know everything all at once, but that was not possible. I had *time* as an essential enemy. Decisions had to be made quickly. With the help of Gene, we chose some type of protocol, knowing that the cells that had escaped into my blood stream were out there, and that even with chemotherapy and radiation, they might win the battle.

Gene and I read as much research as possible. I tried committing the turgid language of my original pathology report to heart. Still, we had only a brief interlude to philosophize about the obvious, and move into treatment.

In quick succession, I was *The Girl with the Port, The Girl with No Hair, The Girl Who is Getting Fatter.* The weeks and then months of blood draws, infusions, scans…does one ever come to terms with these intrusions? In that initial phase of my cancer, I felt as if I were suspended on some high precipice, looking down at myself. The fierce intellectual fighting back eventually gave way to a silent acceptance. Silence was my real companion; I met her early in my childhood when my alcoholic father would make my sister and me accompany him to "the store" which was his way of going to a bar in the bad section of town. We were never to speak of it; I would cry from shame, but those were silent tears. Not once in the first seven years of my breast cancer occurrences, did I shed a tear. At the first feelings of sadness, it was as if a turbulent wind would suck all the feeling out of my body; I was a shell, I was a mollusk, I was a tin man of my own making.

2000 to 2005—the years of reprieve, years in which I was nurtured by teaching college students and adults, and bringing 'brown bunny' Maggie-the-poodle into our lives.

A clean mammogram in 2004, and a troubling one in 2005. So, five and a half years of finding one's way back into one's body, of peeling back the onion of fear, and suddenly, a mammogram manifesting 'a snowstorm of DCIS' as described by a surgeon at Sloan Kettering. This time a left -sided mastectomy appeared inevitable. The Amazon would finally lose some of her armor! And the pathology report was maddeningly ambiguous: nothing to virtually classify the tissue as a tumor, but clear lymphatic invasion. After five years of living with ambivalence, the unwanted companion appeared to have taken root.

For me, there was that renewed sense of disassociation, a feeling that the mind would not necessarily triumph over a body under renewed attack. I was not fearful, or depressed, just more like a dog that hears a sound and puts his ears up, way up! Chemotherapy was advised and, once again, the regimen was accepted.

Winters can be dark and dank in the Northern Adirondacks, but it was in that wet winter of 2005–2006 that I joined a unique breast cancer survivor group in Burlington, Vermont, on Lake Champlain, Dragonheart Vermont, a boating group devoted to women and men in all stages of breast cancer. From 2006 onward, I learned the rigorous strokes of dragon boating, challenging my mind and body and gaining the camaraderie of other breast cancer survivors. I learned to be comfortable in my body, and humbled by those women whose physical journeys were halted by the ubiquitous disease of breast cancer.

It was in early June of 2007, as our coach had us doing heats on The Charles River in Boston, that I had a significant emotional breakthrough. Our boat was in a heat with skilled young men, and their boat felt as if it was floating by us at an unbeatable speed. Coach J. shouted, "You can do it ladies, you're almost there!" It was absurd, it was funny, but oh, so fantastic! I felt the tears welling up, tears that had been locked inside of me for a long time. I felt a spiritual peace and joy that has stayed with me since that day. Did I dismiss the dark companion at that moment? I like to think so.

When breast cancer lesions showed up in my lungs in the winter of 2009, and my new diagnosis was metastatic 4th stage breast cancer, I felt strangely calm. My participation in dragon boating and the continued love and care of my spouse, family and friends, has only deepened my commitment to keeping the unwanted companion at bay.

THE DAY MY LIFE BEGAN TO CHANGE

Carol Germ

I know exactly when it started. It was a sunny day in May of 2003 and I was on my way to hang a bundle of wash on the clothesline. About halfway there, a sharp pain started in my right knee. Looking down, I thought I may have tripped unknowingly on a sprinkler head. This was not the case because there was no sprinkler head even close.

 My next thought was to get those clothes hung to dry and then just walk out this cramp or whatever it was in my right knee. I hobbled to the clothesline and literally had to crawl back the fifty feet to the house. The only bright spot going for me now was the fact those clothes did get hung.

Not being able to recall a recent injury, there was no reason this should be happening. The sudden onset and constant pain I was experiencing would need a visit to a Doctor. Since it seemed to be bone related going to see an orthopedic Doctor was my first choice. I knew such a Doctor personally so called and was able to get an appointment for three days out.

Three days later, a strange thing had happened. My severe knee pain was gone but my right shoulder was now starting to hurt. I decided to keep my appointment as I still did have joint pain, except now it was in my right shoulder. I tried to tell the Doctor this but he did not listen and ordered an x-ray of the right knee and told me it looked fine and should not be causing me any further pain. I asked again about the pain that had now moved to my right shoulder and he said this was probably nothing to worry about and I had most likely "stretched a muscle."

The visit to see my friend the orthopedic Doctor was not a total failure. While in the waiting room of the clinic, I read a story in an old magazine about the actress Kathleen Turner. She had been suffering with a similar painful condition that also caused her to have extreme fatigue for over a year. She had been to see several Doctors regarding these symptoms but no one had given her a diagnosis and they seemed to believe some of this was "in her head." They also felt she was probably working too much and just stressed out. I remember thinking how can this be happening to someone with plenty of money and probably good access to Doctors. She was eventually diagnosed with Rheumatoid Arthritis.

What I didn't know at the time was this was also going to happen to me. Luckily, the time for me from initial symptoms to diagnosis was four months. During this time, I would continue to have severe, rotating joint pain that would last about three days in any given area, then give me three days when I would be completely pain free. When the pain would return, it would attack a different joint. This rotating pain made it through all joints including my hands, jaw, ankles and toes. Just one area would be affected at a time and it did feel at times I was imagining the severe pain because when it was not there I would feel fine and all joints moved well.

There was some help I received from my gynecologist when she prescribed a decreasing dose of prednisone. This was a magic drug for me as it worked well to decrease the inflammation and soon my pain would be gone. I realized soon that this must be some type of arthritis and I made an appointment to see a rheumatologist. That appointment was three months away and during the wait time I would suffer pain if I was not taking prednisone during the flare ups. Doctors do not like to prescribe prednisone on a long-term basis because of the side effects but it was the only thing that even began to help relieve the pain.

My first visit to see a rheumatologist was interesting. He was a chatty guy who spent time with his patients, mostly discussing his philosophies of life. He did tell me I had the classic symptoms of a type of rheumatoid arthritis that could continue and get worse or it may just go away as suddenly as it had began. Of course, what I heard was that it was "going away" and I would no longer need to deal with these symptoms of extreme pain.

This did not happen and now eight years later I am still learning to live with RA. I definitely wanted to deny that I had a chronic illness for years and when I had times of feeling good I would think, "I beat it." Then I would make plans to do things with lots of energy and enthu-siasm for life. After many times of getting "burned" by too much activity, I backed off and started to pace differently. Rheumatoid Arthritis can be painful but this disease also causes feelings of fatigue. This is a big discouragement for people who have had plenty of energy to be active and keep up with the responsibilities of life.

After the diagnosis comes the treatments that are not without side effects. It is a trial and error combination to find what works best for most people. Then it is hoping the treatments will keep your symptoms to a minimum so you can continue contributing to society and be fairly free of pain.

There is also the experience of relating to the health care workers on a continuing basis because you are now a person with a chronic disease. The appointments seem to come around too soon and you hope that the doctor visits become more than "cattle calls" as you see the same providers throughout the year. I have had the experience of seeing six rheuma-tologists. I would say only one of those was a person who seemed as pleased to see me as I was to see her. She moved her practice and it was time again to find a different doctor. So goes life with a chronic illness and the most you can hope for is your health providers are knowl-edgeable and willing to listen.

For me, learning to live with a chronic illness or a terminal illness a person, must develop insight and know life is really about the moments. We have moments in the present and the moments of memories from the past that make up our lives. All other time is lost and the fu-ture may be well planned but it may also throw us a curve ball. If we enhance our moments, life will have a sense of joy to it.

BREAST FRIENDS FOREVER

Adele L. Bergstrom

I quit wearing a bra when I was seventeen. Gloria Steinem gave me permission. Sitting bra-less at my first Women's Lib meeting, legs crossed, ankle over knee, dragging on a Camel cig-arette, I felt masculine and free. That same year a relative took me aside at a family gathering to warn me what gravity would do to my pendulous breasts, but I refused the bra she offered to buy.

When my breasts first sprouted, I'd strapped them in with a wide belt because they didn't fit the tomboy roles I played with my brother. Still, guided by six older sisters, I eventually learned to embrace them, even like them. Heavy and drooping, they never stood at attention yet they inspired admiring glances from men of all ages. Even as a hippie in rough-hewn clothes, I drew catcalls from construction workers that I secretly welcomed.

My breasts took on new meaning—and new shape—when I became a mom, providing the sole sustenance for three babies during their first six months' of life. The day our last baby stopped nursing, I cried. When our older son caught a glimpse of them as I bent to tie his shoe he joked, "They look like two big teardrops!" Our daughter sketched a picture of me with pink crayon on scrap paper, a large, rounded "W" for my breasts. I laughed and hugged her. If chil-dren had hastened such disfigurement, it was worth it!

The year I turned fifty, my periods ended. I signed up for a spring class in Mindfulness Meditation. Outside, the ground was thawing. Inside, the sun shone through the windows of the simple studio as we sat on our mats and contemplated eating an orange. I thought, too, about how my body would fare in menopause.

Halfway through the course, I went in for my annual mammogram. Over the years, x-rays had revealed lumps. Twice, I'd had tissue removed for closer examination with benign results. The phrase "lumpy breasts" became familiar. This time, something had changed.

"The doctor wants to take another look," the technician informed me. A follow-up ultra-sound confirmed suspicious calcifications. A needle biopsy was scheduled.

On the drive to a water-themed motel for our kids' spring break, I slumped in the front seat, reading an essay by Barbara Ehrenreich detailing her experience with breast cancer. What would my story be if this were my prognosis?

A few days later, I got the call. The biopsy revealed ductal carcinoma in situ or DCIS, con-fined to a milk duct in my right breast. It could be removed easily with a lumpectomy, the doctor assured me, followed by six weeks of radiation.

Six weeks? Our son was graduating from high school in June.

I scheduled the lumpectomy for late April at a major university hospital that spans both banks of the Mississippi. Using ultrasound, a technician on the *east* bank would insert a guide wire through the nipple to direct the surgeon. Wire in place, I'd go to the *west* bank for surgery.

I arrived alone for the lumpectomy. The same day procedure required minimal recovery. I wanted my husband to be with our kids when they got home from school. The technician deftly inserted the wire. "Looks good," she said, handing me a wrinkled robe to cover the back of my gaping hospital gown. Gathering up my belongings, I moved to the lobby to wait for my ride.

A middle-aged man in a medi-van arrived. Clutching my robe, I allowed him to take my arm as I climbed into the passenger seat. He regaled me with tales of botched procedures on the drive across the river. "The clip on my bile duct didn't hold...Christ, I was in pain!" Climbing out of the van, I imagined a twilight zone of freaks of which I was now a part, witness the wire protruding from my breast.

The surgery went fine—or so I thought. A day later, the surgeon called. Because the margins around the calcifications weren't "clean," he needed to remove more tissue. Two-thirds of the breast would be gone by then. He recommended a mastectomy, but I could choose.

I decided to switch clinics, selecting a world-renowned breast center across town that offered surgery, chemotherapy, breast reconstruction along with both physical and mental therapy, a library and coffee served in fine china while you waited.

Once I'd accepted the loss of my breast, I moved forward meekly, anxious to be done with doctors, hospitals and medi-vans. Mentally, I detached from my friend, the right breast that had been with me for forty years, the one I'd preferred through decades of lovemaking and nursing.

One May day it was there, the next, gone, along with the sentinel lymph nodes under my arm. I awoke to a large bandage covering the place it had been. I spent days in a morphine-induced stupor, wrestling with harrowing nightmares that dredged up odd snippets of childhood: an eighty acre farm with a house of horrors set up on the back forty. A choir assembled along a narrow ledge that dripped black goo. The ominous danger of being sucked into a deep muddy hole or worse—falling off the ledge into an abyss. Sobering up, I knew I had faced death.

In early September, I started chemotherapy, braced for the infamous side effects of nausea and low energy. A few days later, my husband loaded up our son in a U-Haul and drove him to college on the coast, leaving me with our two younger children and my maimed body. I sat at the kitchen table, sipping green tea, gazing out into the back yard.

Out of nowhere, a pit the size of a shallow grave had opened up in our garden that summer, sucking in Frisbees and the occasional athletic shoe. Our best guess was it was part of an old foundation. The younger kids feared it and I'd become obsessed with filling it.

The anti-nausea meds made me feel strangely competent and strong. I bought bags of dirt and a few perennials on sale at the garden store and lugged them home. I set to work, jerking the bags across the yard. The exertion hurt, but the bodily insults I'd endured over the past months only fueled my determination to fill this maddening eyesore. I finished plugging the pit in less than three hours. The headiness I felt—being able to fix this mysterious blot on my own—brought sublime satisfaction along with release of the bottled-up anger I hadn't acknowledged.

I live mostly pain-free now, save for the scar tissue that sometimes flares up when I flex my pectoral muscle. Reconstruction surgery gave me a new faux breast, complete with a nipple that looks authentic but has absolutely no feeling and can never replace my old friend.

My repair in the garden appears permanent. The perennials grow profuse in the new dirt. My hair has grown back dark, thick and curly. I have every reason to believe I made the right choices. Still, I wrestle with the loss. My breast is gone, along with all it represented—our shared history, growing up together. Despite the plastic surgeon's best effort, that can never be replaced.

TERESA KLEINSCHMIDT

Wearing shorts, sandals and a t-shirt, I shiver in twelve-degree weather. My two companions joke about dissociation and survival. The wind coughs its frigid breath as we wait to jump into Lake Minnetonka, on New Year's Day, 2012. Jumping into icy water on the first of the year has intrigued me since I first saw reports of it, when I was in elementary school. "I gotta do that!" whizzed through my brain and caught in the cells that hold my memory.

Fast-forward thirty-five years as I try to smile and fake excitement. The audio of my nighttime conversations haunt me, even in the bright morning. Last night, my shadow didn't let me sleep. It taunted me with thoughts of rescue teams retrieving my body from the icy waters, because my blood sugar plummeted due to the shock of the temperature change. Images of my bloody feet, permanently numbed into neuropathy, troubled me because I always worry when my feet get cold. And as always, I am surrounded by the hum of questions about whether by body will need more or less insulin or carbohydrates, because I am unsure how this new experience will affect my body.

Twenty-nine years ago, my pediatrician diagnosed me with Type I Diabetes. An autoimmune disease, my body attacked my pancreas, instead of the invading virus. As a result, my pancreas stopped producing insulin. Insulin allows the body's tissues and organs to access blood sugar and utilize its energy. If insulin is absent, the sugar stays in the blood stream and toxins are created as the body tries to rid itself of it. Thus, all the complications of diabetes: Poor circulation and neuropathy in the feet and hands; Kidney damage, possibly resulting in kidney failure; and Retinopathy, which at its worst results in blindness.

Because my mother was dying of lung cancer at the time of my diagnosis, my family was unable to absorb any more trauma. I was on my own from the first. Hearing the term diabetes, reminded me of the stories of my paternal aunt. Spoken quietly, my mother used words like "coma" and "miscarriage" when describing the few times my aunt had been pregnant. I immediately swallowed my tears and went to the hospital for four days. Smiling nurses administered insulin while informing me I would be doing this on my own at home. I took classes about complications, diet and infections. My dad attended sporadically, and then only interrupted to ask questions about my mother's cancer. "If she ate more vegetables, would that improve her outcome?" It was impossible for him to focus on the disease affecting his daughter.

Dropped off at the clinic's entrance, I would attend weekly appointments alone. During one visit, a nurse told me that I would never be able to wear an engagement ring, because it might get caught on something and injure my finger. "Diabetics don't heal like other people. Infections are dangerous." I returned from that appointment and told my mother. She scoffed and told me I could wear whatever ring I wanted. That was the last time she would reassure me and correct the crazy, inaccurate information I would receive throughout my life. Almost six weeks to the day of my own diagnosis, my mother lost her fight to an even scarier disease.

Enter my shadow. Because support evaded me, I swallowed my fears and confusion. I couldn't endure the emotional message that if I didn't follow the strict medical regiment prescribed; ugly, painful complications would arise. So my shadow emerged through a smoky haze, revealing ugly teeth and a scarred face. An unwanted companion, I avoid its presence at all costs. It can trick me into listening, making me believe that it provides only truth. Springing out of nowhere, it brings up worries of comas and neuropathy. Minutes before giving a speech or boarding a plan, I hear murmurs of low blood sugars and insulin going bad. It catches me most often with guilt. If I haven't been testing blood sugars or giving insulin in a timely manner, it reminds me that diabetes could destroy my life at any moment.

In the movie, *A Beautiful Mind*, Paul Bettany plays Charles, the friend created by John Paul Forbes' psychotic mind. Through most of the movie, he portrays a caring, friendly roommate. In fact, the viewer believes he is a real person. Instead, Charles is a hallucination formed by schizophrenia, an illness Forbes fights as he succeeds in his academic career. I question how I might transform my shadow into something a bit lighter, one able to converse and negotiate. It could represent my fears, but also present them in a more practical, adaptable manner. We could talk about the sensation of frozen feet and how different it is from a foot with neuropathy. We could acknowledge that everyone has "floaters" and that they don't mean a precursor to blindness. Allowing my shadow to become a friendly sort, would require me to stare into the smoke and read the messages underneath. I would have to decipher truth from folklore and acknowledge the statistical probabilities of amputations, dialysis and seizures.

From the beginning, I buried any thought that brought me fear. If the possibility of being "sick" existed, I didn't want to know about it. I quarantined it to become fodder for my shadow. If I could avoid experiencing terror, my shadow had permission to show me glimpses of my anxieties later on. Part of this bargain involved avoiding triggers that my shadow regurgitated almost immediately. I learned to benignly ignore the disease, justifying it as self-sacrifice. From diagnosis, I made diabetes as unobtrusive as possible. I pretended I could be 'normal" without bothering people with my treatment. This meant delaying injections and avoiding blood tests, to sidestep the possibility of disturbing others with the sight of a syringe or blood. I reassured friends that we could lengthen our bike ride without stopping for a snack, and prayed that my low blood sugar would occur towards the end. These little missteps affected my overall health but if the shadow could keep its side of the bargain and limit its reminders, I would keep mine. In the last few years, however, my shadow has been gambling with this agreement. I lose sleep and lack the enjoyment of new activities because of the whispers of worry that occur more frequently.

My shadow is insisting that I face that my lack of precision, over almost thirty years, cannot be ignored. I begin to face a stronger probability that any moment, my doctor will announce a complication has been identified. In order to avoid provoking my shadow further, I must develop a friendship with my uneasiness of this disease. Like a companion who continues to aggravate me into observing its presence, diabetes must be faced and managed. This friendship will require a new bargain of openly prioritizing my treatments and provide me with the possibility of health, both mental and physical. "Greetings, mi amigo."

BETTY GRABLE LEGS

Kristine Zimmer Orkin

It was a beautiful summer evening and I was on my way to meet him. Descending slowly the two flights of stairs, through an atmosphere hushed with anticipation, I walked to where he lay waiting for me. The setting before me so beautiful and peaceful that surely I had to be dreaming, it paled in comparison to the heart of my destination. My eyes focused only on the man I loved.

The night air blew warm and the sheet hung loose on his body, covering his torso down to mid-thigh. Drawing closer, I noticed his lower limbs left exposed and smiled to myself.

There they are. Those unmistakable Betty Grable legs.

"They're my identifying feature," he'd once told me when I questioned the strange epithet. "My mother says that even as a baby, I had beautiful legs. Recognizable legs that distinguished me from others. My legs portray character. Mom says they're 'Betty Grable legs.'" A declaration issued with pride and self-esteem.

Betty Grable legs? Was he serious? What mother brands a young boy with a label like that, comparing his features to those of a 1940s pin-up model? Even more curious, what boy—now grown man—not only admits to that moniker, but embraces it? Even brags about it?

Nonetheless, his celebrated gams became a private little joke between us, a topic of continual appraisal and subject to intimate teasing. Admittedly, his shapely appendages often caught my attention, especially in the early stages of our relationship. I was drawn to them each time he donned a pair of running shorts. Skimpy apparel during the 1970s and '80s, the shorts barely covered one's bottom, leaving legs unrestricted and noticeably unclothed.

His were strong legs, short and muscular. Fleshy thighs with well-rounded calves that tapered into strong slim ankles. Betty Grable-like, to be sure. Any resemblance to the blonde bombshell ended there.

Well-exercised legs, accustomed to daily jogs on a well-planned circuit around town. Legs that delighted in cycling jaunts of fifty miles or more on sunny weekends, less when our kids were in tow. He enjoyed strolling any golf course, any time, as often as possible—trudging uphill to tee shot areas, hiking across long and sometimes winding fairways, maneuvering cumbersome sand traps.

His were long-suffering legs that endured monotonous household chores—the lifting of heavy boxes and furniture, climbing stairs from basement to attic, up and down repeatedly, toting baskets of laundry or miscellaneous paraphernalia. Legs resilient to steady pacing back and forth, pushing a lawnmower through a backyard of overgrown grass or navigating a grocery cart through heavily congested food store aisles.

Legs that were sturdy enough to support one child in his arms and another on his shoulders for the duration of a Christmas parade; limber enough to play "horsey" in the evening with wild young cowboys; comfortable enough to balance sleepy children as he read to them or rocked them at the end of the day, then carried them upstairs to their beds and knelt with them to pray.

Mystifying legs that could be fast and sure when it came to sports, offering challenging competitions to growing sons on baseball and soccer fields, basketball and tennis courts. Those same legs abruptly mutated into two left feet on the dance floor, composure and rhythm returning only during slow romantic tunes as we held each other tight.

I took a full minute to gaze upon his face, then knelt and kissed him gently on the mouth. His chest cushioned my head as I embraced him. Nearly bursting with overwhelming love, I never wanted to let go. In the stillness of the moment, my mind conjured up scenes of our life together: The day we met. Falling in love. Our endless conversations about things of great import and coveted talks about nothing at all. The celebrations, the arguments, and the passion we put into both. The children we had created and nurtured. The family bond we cherished.

Slowly my senses came alive as I returned to the moment at hand. A gentle breeze and dip in temperature signaled oncoming nightfall. Sounds of dusk hummed in my ears—birds harmonizing in nightly melodic rituals; solitary insects buzzing close by, looking for one last meal among the flower petals; gnats swarming in angry black clouds around my head; children's laughter squealing in the distance; assorted fragrances filling my nostrils and stirring memories of other summer nights.

My knees began to ache. The realization that I was prostrate on hard concrete interrupted my reverie. With head still upon my husband's chest, I slowly opened my eyes and spotted the lone policeman several yards down, re-routing cyclists on the bike path. The same path where my love and I were sharing a private moment. Glancing upward, I stared at the onlookers leaning over the rails of the street-level bridge above. They stared back, taking in the scene below. Then gentle hands, one on my back and one on my elbow, helped me to my feet. I panned my surroundings. People gathered quietly off to the side, some sitting on the grass, some standing. Normal folks, out for a bike ride on a pleasant summer evening. All of them gazing in my direction, a look of guarded expectancy on their faces. Paramedics. Police. The coroner's vehicle idling a few feet away. Funny, I hadn't noticed that van or any of these people when I came down the steps to this bicycle path. How long had it been? When did all this commotion happen? A few minutes ago? An hour maybe? A lifetime ago?

~

He'd left earlier than usual for work that morning. An important business meeting was on his mind. Barely sunrise, I lay sleeping as he kissed me goodbye. Now, twelve hours later, not quite sunset, he lies sleeping as I kiss him goodbye.

As the sheet is put in place again, I look one last time at his legs, burning their image into my memory, engraving them on my heart.

The irony of his treasured trademark hit me. Those beautiful legs indeed proved to be his identifying feature.

* * * * *

That was June 13, 2007. Wednesday. A lovely summer evening in Milwaukee, Wisconsin. The temperature warm but comfortable. The sun shining as it started its journey downward toward the horizon. I had just been escorted to the place where my husband died less than an hour before from an apparent heart attack while riding his bicycle on the path that wound through our city and down to Lake Michigan. I was there to identify his body. It's a night I'll never forget, yet there are stretches of time that I don't remember living. It was the longest night of my life, and it happened in an instant.

How does one prepare for your loved one's unexpected death? The only resource I had to draw upon was my faith. The moment the words "I'm sorry; your husband passed away" touched my ears, time stopped and the world emptied.

Just me. Alone with God.

Lord, stay with me. I need You.

He was there. He is still here with me. And I continue to need Him.

He is my strength....

JEANNE MARIE RIESE

Sara and I walked slowly away from the revelry and heat of the Solstice bonfire into the dark night, carrying empty dishes. Snow crunched under our boots and the frigid night air smarted in our lungs. Spontaneously, as if on cue, we both threw back our heads and howled long and loudly, wailing from the depths of our souls as if from a forgotten time.

In my *Life Since Cancer,* I howl loudly at the moon with grief and sorrow.

It was May of 2008, the first evening after my husband Randy was diagnosed with a rare and deadly cancer. In a darkened hotel room, I sat cross-legged on the couch in shock, warmed only by my laptop, agonizing over what was to come, and feeling fiercely protective of my husband who had finally escaped into sleep.

During the day, incessant calls from family and friends had replayed the devastating news time after time. Cancer was the insidious unwelcome evil invader. The cancer would die or my husband would die; the two could not coexist. On that fateful night, confronted with a future of dark uncertainty, and on the brink of a new and unexpected journey with my husband, I started writing the first few stanzas of *The Epic Love Poem*:

> Be fierce, My Love, be fierce.
> Life as we know it, is done.
>
> The battle to the death has begun.
>
> The castle watch failed—
>
> The wall was scaled.
>
> No time to be sad,
>
> No time to be mad,
>
> For the enemy is here;
>
> it's very, very bad.

> Be fierce, My Love, be fierce.
>
> The Greatest Battle of all
>
> Is to keep your Spirit tall
>
> And never fall.
>
> Your flesh may be devoured
>
> And your defenses cower
>
> But your Spirit must tower.
>
> Do what you love,
>
> Love what you do.
>
> It's time to be true.

Be true, My Love, be true.

Channel your fears,

Brush away my tears.

Use your charms

To gather me gently into your arms.

Cherish our time

As so very, very fine.

As I drafted *The Epic Love Poem*, I listened to Randy breathe, just as I would listen to him breathe on many, many, sleepless nights, praying for the next breath, until 734 nights later my best friend died in my arms as I whispered yet more messages of love.

In my Life With Cancer, I cherish the living, I honor the dead, and I write.

My husband and I tried very hard to focus on what we most valued: Family, Friends, God, and Nature. Our brothers and sisters, nieces and nephews, parents, and cherished friends had been, and continued to be our center. I am forever grateful for the parents and teachers of our four of young nieces in southeast Wisconsin who would arrange for Randy and me to spirit the girls out from their classrooms so they could skip and run to the park with Randy for a few cherished hours during the short visits we could manage during Randy's last two years of life. The photos and memories of pure joy, giggles and unrestrained laughter, of swinging high, playing on the monkey bars, racing to give Uncle Randy the biggest bear hug, will always be treasured.

For Randy's last birthday, his fiftieth, we had two parties—one for family in the south, and one for family and friends up north. Life was good. Every single brother, sister, in-law, niece and nephew, all thirty-two, from all around the country came to Randy's last Thanksgiving in 2009. We gave thanks that day. Our cup was overflowing.

In my *Life After Cancer*, I spend more and more time with family and friends, less and less time worrying about things that cannot be changed and decisions already made.

I now covertly watch elderly couples and guess how long they have been together—husbands and wives who finish each other's sentences, who still hold hands and kiss exactly on target without even looking. I am not jealous, but I do grieve that my chance to grow old together with my husband was cruelly stolen.

On early summer moon-filled evenings like the one on which Randy died, I often walk down the steps of our cabin to stand on the dock that juts out into the lake. There I listen to the loons and crickets, gaze at the stars reflected in the waters, and commune with nature and my thoughts. As I sort through the complexities of loss, I embrace the good things I learned from all the people I loved who died before me. The deaths left voids, but good lessons and memories too.

From my late husband, I learned to view life's cup as half full rather than half empty. From Mother, I learned to appreciate beauty and grace. From Father and Grandmother, I learned to value hard work, generosity, and education. From my mother-in-law, I learned quiet contemplation and passionate love.

In my *Life After Cancer*, I commune with those who went before me, still sharing their love and wisdom.

Birth, life, cancer and death are complex and messy. Just as birth is awe-inspiring, being in the presence of death is an honor, overwhelming in its power and finality. Just six weeks before my husband died, I was at my Mother's bedside in her hospital room, helping her to listen to piano concertinos on my iPod. Suddenly doctors raced into her room, knowing before we did that Mother's heart was giving out. I held Mother's hands and calmly told her I loved her as she silently suffered a massive heart attack, her whole body tense, hands clinging to mine, eyes huge and watery. Stubbornly living life her way to the end, Mother belied doctors' predictions of minutes to live and held on a few more hours. By then, she could die in peace, cocooned in the midst of her grown children.

I met Kelly Culhane, who lost her battle with breast cancer, through her mother when Bernadette attended a class for cancer patients and caregivers on *The Mysteries of Life After Death*. Kathy, the only surviving cancer patient from the class, is adamant that she will not die alone, that she has a bed large enough so her friends can lie next to her during her fast approaching final days. We will honor her request.

In my *Life With Cancer*, I honor the death process by being fully present and respectful.

Twenty months after my beloved husband's death, the Dark Companion lingers, still unwelcome, its impact profound. The icy cold river of grief and sadness still runs swiftly and deep.

At the same time, my tolerance for ignorance, meanness, and greed is gone. I embrace people of compassion, generosity, and grace. I devote a large part of my life to quiet contemplation and helping others; for writing, painting, sculpting, and listening to music; for hugs and hand-holding; for passion and love.

Ultimately, the only meaningful way for me to honor those who have gone before me and those who battle on, is to embrace life in the here and now, to be wholly present, to live fully and love enormously.

UNINVITED GUEST

Linda Kirchmaier

One day last year I found
Ms. Big C hiding in my house
by my front door
she had taken residence.
Unwelcome guest.

Necessary to excise her hiding place
in case she brought relatives.

Surgeon said none were found.
If she had babies too small for the naked eye
they were expelled along with the hiding place.

Threatening to unnerve
Did any go visiting elsewhere?

Now the game becomes making my house
an undesirable neighborhood for their residence
and a conducive neighborhood for my wholesome friends
While learning to live
with unanswerable questions.

Lately, Ms. C's ghost has been
lurking in the shadows leaving hauntings
when news arrives of another called home.
She starts her un-choreographed dance
lighting up touch points as she pirouettes

leaving behind
more unanswerable questions.

Looks like it's time to further...
tidy up my house.

KEITH JOHNSON

Upon arrival of my cancer illness, there was a ridiculous collision of illogical and even comedic events. Fifteen years later, I still clearly remember these events. Fifteen years later, I still ponder the significance of these events. But the impression of these events is like an indecipherable Rorschach inkblot image. I simply cannot make sense of these events.

Coming to terms with my dark cancer companion is such a personal experience that I question whether I can provide any road map to help someone else navigate the experience. I'm convinced that illness, like love and death, is too terribly personal of an experience to offer up as guidance.

My story began with the stunning diagnosis. My wife fainted. I had a stage IV head and neck cancer. I had discovered a golf-ball-sized lump in my neck. This lump appeared, literally, overnight. My own emotions conjured up the poet Emily Dickinson's lines:

"After great pain, a formal feeling comes. The Nerves sit
ceremonious, like Tombs...."

The recommended treatment was surgery and radiation. The prospects were dubious. The Mayo Clinic doctors were officious and very helpful, but made no grand promises. I also visited a number of homeopathic doctors, along with exploring (and eventually using) alternative cancer treatments in Mexico. One of the holistic doctors, when I told her of my squamous cell carcinoma, declared a bit too honestly: "Ooooh, that's a killer." Thanks for the dead-on assessment, doctor.

After the initial diagnosis, my wife and I drove the forty miles home in stunned silence. As I drove the quiet final miles to our home, the silence was shattered by a morning dove splatting against our windshield. The dove was stuck, entangled in the windshield wiper right in front of me. We drove on, still speechless. Seconds before this smash I'd been pondering my mortality. Now I was staring at a dead dove, flopping in the wind right before my eyes. Should I turn the windshield wipers on? Doing so would send bloody bird streaks across the windshield. I half-heartedly calculated the chances that the dove might fly off the windshield if I turned the wipers on ... or it might not, leaving the view of a dead dove flopping back and forth across our horrified view.

I did nothing. My wife said nothing. A few torturous miles later, the dead dove mercilessly flopped free from the windshield wiper's clutch. I wondered—hoped really—that this dead dove's life was a sacrifice for mine. Such were my desperate yearnings.

My cancer had metastasized from my tonsil to the lymph nodes in my neck. I was warned that I might have my tongue surgically altered and my jawbone sliced apart in a hinge-like fashion, if they found more invasive cancer. If this was done, my speaking ability would be seriously affected. Since I was a school teacher, I pondered my future as an object of ridicule by ruthless adolescent students.

Despite eight hours of invasive throat and neck surgery (clinically termed "neck resection, which removed my neck muscle and left a "T" shaped scar on the side of my neck"), it wasn't until after the surgery that I learned that my speech capabilities were preserved. Once that surgical crisis had passed, my four-year-old daughter Maria pronounced the surgery a success by observing: "well, at least you can still whistle."

Not only was my ability to whistle in limbo, but another bodily function, I soon learned, was temporarily compromised. Post surgery, I was in the hospital for ten days. Since my throat and neck were the source of surgery, I ate nothing. I'd had a tracheotomy; so I could not eat, could not talk, and certainly had no need to...well, poop. But this adventure was soon to come.

After ten days of not eating, it was finally time to take my first poop. This, I thought, should be an interesting experience. I sat down, applied the necessary pressure, and "shwe-e-e-e-e-z-z-e." Nothing. I was pressure-less. My tracheotomy hole was wheezing, releasing whatever miniscule internal pressure I could muster. I quickly figured out that my plan B was for me to plug my tracheotomy hole with my finger, and by doing so, muster enough pressure to achieve the (ahem) end result. Those results were negligible, but in the short term, I'd devised my own "press-here-to-poop" strategy.

My first hospital walk, a few days after surgery, was also filled with ignominy. My wife and the nurse accompanied me on my first post-surgical steps. My catheter bag was also along for the ride. I'd never had a catheter before, so I was a little confused by its freely swinging presence just south of my knees. I couldn't yet talk, so I could only point to the dangling catheter bag and mime in bewilderment. "Is this right?" It most definitely was not, and the embarrassed nurse quickly secured the bag and relieved my nagging, tugging discomfort.

My ominous thoughts on mortality were leavened by these comical episodes. I could still whistle (didn't feel like it though...), I had to patiently wait until one orifice healed before another one could operate. I now knew that a catheter bag should be attached and not dangle freely. I learned to desperately hope, so much that I hoped that dead dove on my windshield was a good sign. I also learned to pray.

Amidst this flurry of confusing, ridiculous events, one moment of crystal clarity still looms, fifteen years later. My surgery was on a Monday morning at St. Mary's Hospital in Rochester, Minnesota. My fate and the extent of the invasive surgery was unclear. Would I have a jaw? Would I have a tongue to speak? Would I die? My wife and two close friends were a consoling presence during the tedious wait before surgery. Once my number was called, I said goodbye to them and was wheeled away to a pre-surgery holding area. It was here I reached a stark conclusion: I was totally helpless. Whatever was about to happen was completely out of my hands. Quick on the heels of that realization came an unmistakable peace. More than that, it was a peaceful *presence*.

Coming to terms with my "dark cancer companion" was, and still is, crystallized in that long moment. I've told few people of my experience with this peaceful presence, since it was an utterly personal experience. Any attempt at describing this experience makes it trite. But it was clear to me: I was helpless and I was helped; I was anxious and I was calmed. I felt it. I experienced it. I'll never forget it.

I still chuckle and marvel at the comedy of errors that occurred throughout my illness. I shudder at the scars of the surgery and I still suffer the lingering effects of the radiation. But foremost and forever after, I treasure that single moment when I was allowed to feel that peaceful presence so clearly.

CANCER, MY ALLY

Rachel Nelson

Blood and bone.
I look down, sea of bright red.
My feet are engaged in earthly matters
of life and death.
Am I a dried-up old fencepost
in this flood
or can I still tap the red root
for life
blood
and bone?

The call came on New Year's Day, 1996: "We have a diagnosis of invasion, Rachel. Happy New Year." It was my blunt gynecologist. She had not trusted previous test results, given my condition: barely over 100 pounds, almost constant vaginal bleeding, abdominal pain, palpable mass.

What poured over me was immense relief. Finally, a name to what had been going on for a year. That's how long it had taken me to see a doctor. At that moment, I stepped out of denial and into life. My vision cleared.

My gynecologist recommended the surgeon she would trust, if it were her. "If he agrees to take medical assistance," she added.

He did. And so the gifts began.

A friend who had heard the news called me to recommend a hands-on healer/psychic. At our first meeting, Nancy told me two things: first, she recommended writing a poem to my uterus before my operation, to say goodbye and thank you. This was an enormously emotional experience for me. I thanked my uterus for giving its life to save mine.

Secondly, Nancy, whose gifts include seeing emotional issues that the body is carrying, said to me, "I see a buried child inside you. I have the feeling that if we work together more, we will work with this buried child."

Before my operation, a friend who had come with me to many diagnostic appointments, watching my legs shake in waiting rooms, gifted me with a hands-on healing. During this healing, she said that she saw a bear when she touched my abdomen. When she saw that bear, she knew it would be all right.

The night before I went into hospital, I got out of bed and stomped around in a circle, singing wordless notes while shaking my pill bottle. I didn't know how to pray.

After the operation, my partner was in the hospital room when I woke up. I told her that I felt better than I'd felt in a year—no pain, mass gone! Then I confided that I also felt a bit afraid to go back to sleep.

"Do you remember what the Doctor said to you as you were going under, about the results of your scan?" No, I said. "He said your scan showed a much bigger involvement than they had thought." Obviously, some part of me remembered. From then on, I focused on what was in front of me: healing from the surgery.

On one of my first walks around the hospital halls, I found my way to the chapel. I sat down and started to cry. This was a Catholic hospital, and one of the nuns walked in and asked me if I would like to pray. I shook my head. She asked if she could pray for me. I nodded, unable to speak. I still remember this woman's kindness.

I remember also my surgeon's kindness, checking in on me much more than he needed to during my hospital stay. Saying "just heal; we'll talk about things when you get out."

After my release, my partner and I were in his office. My chart was in his hands. First he went through a few facts which told my partner, who had been doing her research, just how bad it was. I was oblivious to this, until I noticed tears in my doctor's eyes. He cleared his throat; then said, "I never say never to anyone." What luck—to have a surgeon wise enough to know that he couldn't know. His words left me room to recover.

From then on, I had an internal gyroscope that gave me clear signals as I navigated my treatment choices. I surprised myself by saying yes to radiation therapy, even gaining weight during that treatment. I found a wonderful dietary advocate who schooled me on macrobiotic eating and periodically tested my body to see what foods would be helpful.

All during my radiation therapy, I wore a shirt to the clinic with a bear on it, to remind me of the bear spirit my friend had seen. "It's a mind thing," I told the technicians. They smiled. They got it.

After radiation, I was very clear about chemo. I heard a voice inside me say "chemo will kill you." And I wanted to live! I was writing now, journals, poems, songs, pouring out of me. I wrote now because I couldn't help it.

Just to play the devil's advocate, I asked my doctor, "Could I write on chemo?"

"Well—maybe," he said doubtfully. I declined the chemo, and my doctor said, "That's a reasonable decision."

I knew he thought my decision was based upon wanting quality time for my time left. But doors kept opening for me—I found a body purification technique which I used in lieu of chemo, and I found wonderful art therapies at Minneapolis' Pathways, where I could have free alternative therapies donated by providers every month to assist my healing process.

Most importantly, I was working with Nancy the psychic, doing very deep emotional work. I learned that the body can hold trauma until one is ready to deal with it. Long frozen, I had to take the leap:

> I stand at the edge
> looking down.
> pebble, boot-knocked,
> plummets
> makes no sound
> seems to fall forever
> sweet release.
> My place is here on the edge,

and my stance has as clear a trajectory
as that pebble's fall.
One step back—
or forward—
would be so much easier than this
falling, standing still.

This was my most daring and essential healing act. Working with Nancy, I saw that remaining frozen *was* moving: backwards. So I leapt into this work. My inner child, long
dammed up, began speaking even more through writing and song. At last, I was becoming
acquainted with my long-buried creative self.

I have so many to thank! Today, I thank cancer, my ally, for helping me get back onto my
true life's path.

The Wishing Bone

I hold the fine white bone in my left palm,
feel it thrumming with current
from somewhere I cannot see.
I close my fingers around it.
It pulls me with a strong tug,
and we are walking.
The bone has taken me by the hand.
It is leading me now, down the hill
through the tangle of grasses and dense brush,
heedless of snags and thistles, dragging me along,
down and down,
until we reach a small creek where purple
wildflowers bend over the water
on delicate stems.
We stop.

I know that now is the time to wish it: that which I most desire—
time to speak my creation into being.
I know the white bone gives me this power.
The hot sun bores into the back of my neck.
A fly buzzes, lands on the knuckle
of a finger gripping bone.

This is now:
no more excuses
no more journeys to the wise one.
Now I am she.

MARGARET MANDERFELD

If the "Dark Companion" was a monkey, many clichés come to mind: "Monkey on my back" and "Throwing a monkey wrench into the works" both imply an obstacle or hindrance. Is this how I should look at this new chapter in my life? Looking at illness as a nuisance is like swatting at a mosquito to shoo it away in delusional denial. No, that's too cowardly, and NOT facing it is just monkey business that perpetuates fear!

I remember as a kid playing with "Barrel of Monkeys" a trendy low-tech game where the players link arms of little flat plastic monkeys to form a chain. I also recall feeling it wasn't quite right for the monkeys to just dangle from the crooks of their elbows when they have such talented hands with which to grip. I still liked to play with them into my teen tears when I discovered after my first broken heart that I felt like one of those dangling monkeys, unable to grip, suspension in uncertainty.

Not being able to choose my circumstance in any stage can be like a wobbly plastic monkey chain of events, chains that bind, chains that break, a chain reaction in a chain-link fence with barbed wire.

"As much fun as a barrel of monkeys!" Only now, they're more haunting than those wicked flying creatures from *The Wizard of Oz*, hourglass included! Their creepy portrayal of evil was gestured in their frozen expressions as they came to take the friends away.

I was reminded of that disturbing image in the face of a doctor who wore a crisp white coat and a starched smile as he delivered horrible news. Then I felt like I was cast into the dungeon. Trapped with the hourglass of sand where each grain holds a "what if" or an "if only...."

The sands of time...platitude dunes. And the thought of running out of it too soon renders unwelcome anticipation.

The monkeys from the barrel have a fixed plastic smile, a ready and willing posture and are stuck in a pose. I don't want to be like them. I resist the imposed pose.

Now more than ever I'd like to grip with all of the bones and muscles in my experienced hands, not out of desperation, but rather in a plea for more time, more choices, and less dangling.

I want to feel the freedom of a fragrant fresh air breeze. Seeking freedom from fear leads me to love, where the expression of it lingers beyond breezes. It heals at a deeper level than medicine can reach.

Love is the sustenance that is given and received in a continual and ongoing flow, in a chain of generations.

ANDREA OBERG-MCARDLE

These poems are a response to mental illness. Growing up and watching a number of family members and friends suffer from mental illness, specifically depression, has led me to be extremely aware and interested in the subject. Many falsely believe that depression is something people have control over and that medication and treatment are unnecessary; that people should just "get over it." People need to be educated. Education is power and can save lives. I myself have suffered from Post Partum Depression following the births of my three boys. I sought help and am now in a much better place. Others, I know, have not been so lucky. Some never seek help and live most of their days in darkness, lose everything they have, or worse. Some simply give up, not realizing that hope and healing live within all of us. Sometimes the bravest thing you can do is face your demons, but not necessarily alone. Sometimes the most courageous thing is to humbly admit you need help. Our lives are brief. There are some illnesses that cannot be treated and some accidents we cannot prevent. There is help for mental illness and we're learning more about it every day. Depression is treatable. I feel very fortunate and will forever be thankful for that.

All Consumed

Cross-legged sipping
jasmine tea-
Not knowing if the sun is rising
or setting.
The redundant display of color
is the same either way.
Never knowing directions like he did-
North from south,
East from west
just by a glimpse skyward.
Looking up all I could see was
his face.
If only I could stare at the stars like
everyone else.
And see beauty,
feel wonder for this world.

A lone woman sits in a café
day after day.
Lines creasing her face,
Marks on her back from the
wooden back chair—
The same wooden back chair

day after day.
The same coffee-stained book open
to the same tattered page which
she never reads.
Waiting—
Waiting until the neon
sign flashes *closed* above her head.
Maybe she waits for that sign
so she can glimpse up and see
something else.

Some brightness at the end of her lightless days.

Hatched

Step 1. Cradle the egg in the palm of your hand
Step 2. Insert pushpin into end
Step 3. Rotate egg and insert pushpin into other end
Step 4. Jab pushpin in and out to break up yolk
Step 5. Blow on one end until all of the egg is drained

Job complete. Only the empty shell remains.

Slowly drained by a pinprick—
The killer you never heard coming.
You are left inside—
In the darkness.
The white endlessness—
Smooth on all sides,
stumbling and sliding with
just the tiniest glimpse
of the outside world—
Of how everything actually is.

Depression—
Truly the raw end of the deal.

Trapped and numb,
closed off, but tortured.
Viewing your entire world
in the smallest light.
Never seeing the escape—

Feeling hand over hand,
the boundless shape.
Always searching for
a crevice, a weak spot.
A lost traveler not knowing
which direction to turn,
what place to call home.

Waiting in that carton,
Enclosed, entrapped.
You need someone's hands—
Someone's help,
to make a break—
To fly the coop.
You need a crack—
An opening to emerge.
An opportunity to
take flight.
Waiting for pupils
to constrict,
to see the empty shell
broken at your feet.
Kicking away the debris—
Born again.
Finally seeing
things for what
they truly are—
A thin barrier,
yet structurally sound—
Fragile, delicate,
yet unexpectedly strong.
Not as easily broken
as many may think.

The escapees
smile easily at the thought of
smiling again.
Finally hatched—
Able to make the heavy,
Light.

She Calls Herself Dedra

Good morning,
my name is Jane.
Staring in the mirror—
Again,
my name is Jane.

My world has order.
A paramount type A—
Today has a plan,
a series of
mundane events
equaling up to my
perfectly structured
existence.

Today is a day for
pearls.
A self defining moment
every single time.
Delicate pearls wouldn't
last a day where
Dedra plays.
Luckily she goes
without.

Dedra is the
destruction.
A wrecking ball
battering
my perfect world.
An acute type B—
Completely off the map.
Like wine on a wedding dress;
A stain that will never
come out.

The greasy men
listen closely—
Her whispers of a "sure thing"—
Summoned to her Goth grace.
Her heart a porcelain cold—

Our body a welcome heat—
My extravagant torture.

Living with choiceless guilt
of what she does—
What I do, I suppose.
But when I leave
my heart, my beliefs
leave with me.
The holler of God
turns to white noise—
Nothing more than a
numb, redundant echo.

Hidden beneath blankets,
on the slippery brink of sleep,
contemplating my half-life,
I take a deep breath and
begin to unfold my plea—
My prayer—
The same every night.
My name is Jane.
My name is Jane.
My name is Jane.
Clutching my necklace like a rosary,
pearl after pearl—

Wondering who will wake up in the morning.

Untitled

Directed to the
VIP section
at the hottest spot in town.
The perfect view—
Showing off
from oversized chairs
next to the oversized
picture windows.

A man on the corner,
sign in hand—
Poignant, succinct,

a simple plea for help.
Perched on broken concrete,
scraping grime from
broken fingernails.
Passersby pulling the
turn-away maneuver.
Brutally ignored plus
blatant cruelty,
adding the insult to
the injury.

Staring out
from another world—
Heart pounding—
The beat of drums
playing inside throbs
in my blood.
Designer dress skims the bar,
pressing in on a sculpted body—
The fluid flowing pulse of
satin.

Sipping cocktails,
Biting at politics,
A razor against enamel—
the scrape of plaque.
That killjoy
too harsh for a
Friday night.
Changing subject,
not ready
to reach the roots.
My deliberate avoidance.
Closing the curtain
in this nation of
instant gratification—

Smirking,
I call out—
"This round's on me."

DEATH STALKS MY MOTHER

Lizzy Carney

"I have a problem. I found a lump. They want to do surgery. It might be nothing. Don't come yet."

I couldn't breathe, while trying to comprehend what Mom was saying to me. A lump? Don't come? What was she telling me? Cancer? Long distance is not the next best thing to being there. I put down the phone left with wonderings, what ifs, worrying and waiting while cursing the distance between us. Filled with a longing to be home, to know what was happening, I killed time, not knowing a killer was stalking my mother.

In the darkness, I heard the ringing. Dad could not say the words "breast cancer." He whispered, "They took part of your mother. Please come home."

Mom was in trouble. I was ignorant of the silent silhouette lurking in the shadows of the hospital. I began my journey home. A journey of hope and heart, of fear and frustration, of nightmares and dreams. I did not know what to expect. "They took part of your mother." My head was full of questions as the miles rolled by. Who will help to find the answers? What is ahead for Mom?

Breast cancer. Mastectomy. Who was responsible for these crimes of sickness and pain? I wanted to catch the villain. Stop him from harming my mom. As we were engulfed in the imbalance of diagnosis, treatments and recovery, I needed to eliminate this assassin's threat. I wanted information, doctors and signs of optimism. Mom refused to be a victim of the predator that pursued her. She fought back with faith, hope, love and confidence. Mom had plans and cancer was not one of them. In time, she trusted the verdict. "Cured!" She was a victor over the creeping cancerous criminal.

Confident that justice had been served she moved forward with life: weddings, grandchildren, travels. Life filled her days. We were unaware a persistent and unrelenting shadow remained, plotting to prey on her once again. Slowly, he conspired to reappear.

One day, Mom commented that she was not feeling well. A little pain in her chest and feeling tired. Stress tests, MRIs and consultations uncovered that the insidious scheme was complete. The cancer was back. The deceitful, deviant criminal found no breast to abuse. So he hid behind the bars of her ribs. My mother's surgeon was helpless to bring justice. A football-sized tumor grew silently in the darkness. The oncologists and radiologists teamed up to rightfully overcome the injustice with chemotherapy, radiation and medications. Their caring determination would be the process for justice to diminish and convict the criminal. He had shrunk but kept his hold in the shadows.

While serving his sentence, the hardened criminal learned new assault strategies. Mom's stalker followed her. Irritated that she had beaten him twice, the assassin changed his tactic. She had conquered cancer. His sinister scheme now was to take her piece by piece. Her ability to use her words. Her interests. Her memories!

We lived under the deception that "chemo brain" was the cause for Mom's forgetfulness. But as the years separated her from the treatments, suspicion of the usual suspect lessened.

The stalker was back disguised in the form of a new disease: Alzheimer's.

Like with the cancer, her changes are silent and slow. The stalker is deliberate and unhurried in robbing her of life. He wants more victims, more suffering. He is vindictive toward all who contributed to his earlier convictions. He is stealing my best friend. He deprives, embezzles and burglarizes hope and life. There is no justice for the felony charges of larceny, kidnapping and death. There is no restitution for my tears, loss, sadness or loneliness.

The shadow menacingly loiters constant. I need to eliminate this assassin's threat to my happiness. He is beatable. I will gather my strength and look up at the stars Mom and I so often made our nightly wishes. I will watch the moon rise as we did looking out the window from her bed. I will watch the awe-inspiring cloud formations as imaginary creatures transform overhead. Soon, I will make my wishes and gaze alone, but never will I be truly alone. I will not be threatened by the stalker. He will not get the better of me. Mom is with me in her gifts of love, imagination, courage, elegance, grace and faith. These are gifts from her and will be mine forever.

REMEMBERING MALINDA

Linda L. Klein

When Malinda entered a room, heads turned. Her short, dark auburn hair settled in wisps across high cheekbones. An ever-present smile displayed a row of perfect teeth set against deep rose lipstick. Her soft cowl-neck sweater, the same deep rose as her lips, hid any evidence of Malinda's cancer.

Malinda Verner had Stage IV breast cancer, and she personified the human toll breast cancer takes. She taught me to measure life in moments—not days—never in years. She celebrated that life until the moment she died. To this day, I still resent the comfortable detachment of doctors who viewed Malinda's life as just another statistic in the war on breast cancer. Doctors in white coats at prestigious cancer centers routinely put their feet up on the desk, looked Malinda square in the eye and told her to pray for a miracle while she 'got her affairs in order.' Case dismissed. (This happened. I didn't make it up.)

We met many years ago when Malinda was attending *I Can Cope* classes, and I was researching the book I was writing. We quickly became mutual friends and teachers. She was anxious to share her experiences for the book and to learn from others in her class.

She died less than two years after we met. Yet her haunting presence helped me finish the manuscript for *I Can Cope: Staying Healthy with Cancer.* Shortly after completing that book, the poignancy of Malinda's short life guided my hand through an entire novel that examined the fictional dynamics between a woman like Malinda and an oncologist who lost his personal detachment from his patients and succumbed to his devotion to her. Despite all his self-admonishments, he allowed her into his emotional life—and subsequently suffered the personal and professional consequences of loving something so ephemeral.

Today, years later, her memory still lingers. And I wonder why. Is it because she was so young and vibrant—barely thirty when she died—without a chance at middle age? Or maybe because she represents the millions of women, multiplied by husbands and children and parents, who become a part of this drama?

Breast cancer has a ripple effect, trickling its fear and anger down through every member of the family. Arriving on your doorstep as an unexpected and uninvited guest, it stays. And stays. Sometimes it goes away, and you think it's gone forever. Then, just when you think you can see a future again, it slips in the back door.

I want to share the life-shattering experience of this illness, Malinda would tell me. *And I want my doctor to hear me.* But it was clear that the doctor didn't want to hear her pain. His interest was clinical, not emotional. Topics of fear, loneliness and death were not part of his office visits. The gap between what Malinda was *feeling* and what the doctor was willing to discuss became wider and deeper.

Three months before she died, Malinda and I had lunch at a trendy Minneapolis restaurant. It was her treat. We were celebrating her latest scans, which seemed to show some shrinkage of the tumors in her bones. We lifted our glasses in a toast to the future, but the sound of glass against glass was tentative. I did not want to shatter the moment. We both knew that death had only been delayed, not denied. In most cases, the reality of Stage IV cancer is death. The word "control" replaces the word "cure" in your vocabulary.

Two months before she died, Malinda hosted a summer picnic for her YWCA Encore support group. Her husband had long since abandoned her for a new job in Louisiana, and she was living with a recently-widowed woman friend. Malinda's friend, David, dressed in a tux, was poised to serve frozen daiquiris in fluted champagne glasses. At the time, Malinda was "hooked up," which meant she wore a portable pump that fed non-stop, high-dose chemotherapy through an IV line directly into a catheter near her neck.

But that didn't stop Malinda, former art teacher and eccentric extraordinaire. She tucked the pump into a burgundy leather pouch (to match her outfit), clipped it to her belt, and then hid the tubes under her shirt. I arrived a bit early and found her sweating in the back yard, pulling weeds around the patio so all would be beautiful for the event. When all the guests arrived, the picnic went off without a hitch. Malinda was the perfect hostess, leading the guests to canapés and drinks. Introducing them to David. Taking the time to go one-on-one with each woman. How are you doing? How can I help? From the outside, you would call it a "festive occasion."

If this all sounds too upbeat and normal, let me remind you of the downside. While all the women were mingling outside after lunch, I went to find Malinda to say goodbye. I found her in the living room, alone with David, sobbing in his arms. I was pregnant at the time, carrying the promise of new life. And this beautiful young woman was struggling to hold onto the little bit of life she had left.

One month before she died, weary of the fight, Malinda left her adopted home of Minneapolis to return to Missouri. Home to die. I tried to call her in the hospital, what I now suppose was the hospice wing, but the one phone on her floor always seemed to be in use. I sent a copy of my book and a card. She died before she could read what I wrote about her.

Other Melinda's are out there today—young women finding lumps and being reassured by confident doctors to not be concerned. Many women still trust doctors more than they trust themselves. And that can be a fatal mistake. Malinda's first doctor had never seen inflammatory breast cancer before. The same may be true for many doctors today. He said, "let's watch it." And she did. You know the end of the story. As her illness progressed, she made her doctors more and more uncomfortable. I believe they simply didn't want to deal with the reality of the monster growing inside her, a monster they were powerless to control. Case dismissed.

Malinda's cancer took her to the threshold of life, and she was always keenly aware of how that life could end. She reassessed her values. She came to terms with the end of an already rocky marriage. She kept her artist dreams alive. When she died, she left behind a small leather pouch filled with money she was saving to travel to an Artist's Colony in New Mexico. But time ran out.

Not many days go by when I don't think about Malinda. Recently, walking through a foyer in St. Paul, I could swear I heard her voice. I spun around to find her and came face to face with a stranger. But for a moment—a brief second—she had been with me again, like a dream from which you don't want to awaken. Malinda taught me to measure life in just such moments, though. For that, I am thankful.

HOW I GOT HOPPY

B. J. Johnson

All that summer I compared it to a toothache, the pain in my hips.

It would throb one day, disappear the next. After a hike in the woods, or a long walk with the dog, it would emerge from the depths of my bones, rolling out in rhythmic waves. It would swell and strengthen, commanding attention. Some nights, it would wake me, an evil, unwelcome midnight visitor. I'd kill time staring out at the moonlight, aching and staring, staring and aching.

At the time, the fifty-year mark had just come and gone for me. Too young for this, I thought, whatever "this" was.

Over-the-counter painkillers offered some relief. I bought them in quantity, trying different brands, different strengths, wondering what sort of toll they were taking on my liver or kidneys. The joys of a stiff cocktail were amplified.

Eventually, the pain took up full-time residence, rarely receding, never totally disappearing. My gait changed as I favored the less painful side of my hips. Limping along, distracted by that constant ache, I was finally convinced to visit an orthopedic specialist. We talked through my symptoms, and I got my first introduction to the one-through-ten pain scale. My doctor explained a handful of possible causes and called for x-rays and MRI scans.

Osteoarthritis was the culprit, probably brought on by Femoral Acetabular Impingement, a mystifying bone condition causing the ball of my femur to unnaturally grind away the cartilage in my hip socket. Arthritis, common as it is, was an impossibility for me. I was barely middle-aged and happily in full denial of that. I walked, climbed, canoed, hiked! There was no family history! I was healthy as a horse, I was not overweight, and I hadn't suffered any previous hip injury. Still, in the back of my mind, I dimly recalled a detail about my astrological sign — Sagittarius governs the hips and Sagittarians are prone to diseases and disorders of the hip. So, I thought, it was ill-fated destiny, written in the stars at the moment of my birth.

The grainy, gray, high-tech scanner images told the tale, moderate-to-severe loss of cartilage in both hips. Treatment options from minimalist to draconian were laid out: physical therapy and ongoing pain management, cortisone shots, or surgical hip replacement.

For a few weeks, I went the physical therapy route, stretching, jogging in a pool. I swallowed huge horse pills of glucosamine and chrondroitin sulfate. Neither delivered any noticeable relief. I limped back to the clinic for the cortisone injections.

They readied the tubes and needles. It was an easy, outpatient surgery. A tiny needle prick, a small dribble of blood, and I was on my way. A day later, I went for a hike in some woods near my house. About halfway into the hike, a piercing pain developed in my right hip. I tried limping, even dragging my leg along. The sharp, hot pain was unbearable. It was, I was told later. Probably a cortisone flare, crystals forming and grinding away in soft tissue. Was my cartilage further disintegrating as I limped home through the peaceful woods? After that incident, the pain became ever-present and severe, going from bad to intolerable depending on my attempts at mobility. The doctor prescribed huge doses of ibuprofen. She suggested I try a cane. "I know people your age don't like that, but it really can contribute to pain relief."

I found a cane made by an Austrian mountaineering company. It had a cool look, I thought. I'd cut a dashing figure, as dashing as a fifty-ish guy could be, tottering about, carefully negotiating steps and curbs like an octogenarian.

The singular, tormenting world of chronic pain became morbidly fascinating to me. I'd read about it, but now it was very real, up close and personal. Distracting, disastrous. Strolling, even standing for any length of time, was to be avoided. At parties and family gatherings, I began to feel like a long-forgotten elder, planted in an easy chair far off to the side of the action.

Another round of MRIs revealed the sad reality: *all* of the cartilage had disappeared (gone!) from one hip, and the other wasn't far behind. Bone-on-bone, they said, a painful, hopeless grinding. It's like the rubber on a tire, my doctor explained. When that's gone, the rim grinds along on the road. And, she added, science hadn't yet found any way to surgically put the rubber back on the tire. Total hip replacement, as horrifying as that seemed, was the obvious alternative. The soonest I could have the surgery was two months away, in the dead of a Minnesota winter.

My doctor introduced me to the world of narcotic painkillers. I recall my first few doses, the bizarre, foggy, nodding-off feeling, mixed with a mild sense of bliss, and underneath all of that, the absence of pain! Sweet relief. Too sweet. My tolerance increased, and doses crept up as I chased the numbness. One pill led to one and a half, then two, four, and five were needed. My doctor, experienced in emerging addictions, dispassionately warned me about my consumption, denied my requests for early refills, suggested other, safer pain management techniques.

I was told to use crutches. I thought it would be less embarrassing to use a single crutch than my cane. A crutch—to me—implied a sports injury, a split-second surprise accident that could happen to any vibrant weekend athlete. A cane shouted "long-term, chronic condition," decline and decay. Being told I looked like an oversized Tiny Tim was better than "aging badly, falling apart, old before his time."

At work, a young co-worker teased me, saying with a crotchety, squeaky old voice, "Whatcha got there, a dodgy hip?" I was mortified. Others asked more politely. I perfected a short speech: "I was born with a congenital defect on my femur" (which may or may not be factual, no one knows whether the impingement is there from birth or develops over time). "Now I need surgery." I never used the word arthritis. For a long time, I never said, "hip replacement." When I did, a co-worker tried to cheer me up by saying, "My brother had that. Do you know they literally cut your leg off—dismember the thing! They pull it off to the side then put in the new hardware and re-attach it. How *awesome* is that!? He's fine now."

In November, on a trip to London, I brought my single crutch. At Heathrow, an Indian customs agent sporting an elegant turban greeted me. "Welcome to the United Kingdom," he said. "How did you get hoppy?"

"Excuse me?" I said, not believing I'd heard him correctly.

"Your crutch," he said mildly confused or irritated with my response. "How did it happen?"

I summarized my condition as he stamped my passport. "Okay," he concluded, "hop along now." I got a lot of mileage out of that story.

On New Year's Day, I awoke in a hospital bed. Inside my body were titanium inserts and plastic ball sockets. A miracle of modern medicine, Big Magic from a twenty-first century shaman, a promise that I could walk into the future, pain-free.

MARY SWEERE

I have always considered myself to be a healthy person. Not that I took my health for granted, as our family has always tried to be health conscious, and compared to many others, I felt very fortunate. In mid August of 2007 while visiting California, I noticed a tiny flashing light in the upper corner of my left eye. I attributed it to the bright California sun, but since it had been several years since I had my eyes examined and I desperately needed new glasses, I made a time to visit my optometrist. After a thorough exam, and with an extremely concerned look, he explained he had identified a dark spot behind my left eye. It was behind the retina and adjacent to the optic nerve and that needed further investigation. He was reassuring but took the initiative and made an appointment for me at the Mayo Clinic in Rochester, Minnesota.

Since my background was in health care and I was trained as a registered nurse, I relied on my past knowledge and assumed the best. It would probably be a quick appointment, a diagnosis of some minor but correctable malady, followed by a delicious dinner at one of Rochester's fine restaurants, and we would be on our way home in a few hours. I couldn't have been more wrong. That fateful November appointment changed my life forever, and dramatically impacted our family's life.

For those who may be unfamiliar with the Rochester Mayo Clinic, it is a world- renowned facility specializing in diagnosis, treatment and care of disease. For us, our first visit to the clinic was the beginning of an eye opening, frightening and soul-searching journey.

After checking in and filling out the necessary forms, my husband and I sat in the crowded waiting area observing how many other patients were suffering from various eye conditions and we were filled with a great sense of empathy for them. When I was employed by Steele County Public Health Service, I learned first hand from my former clients that sight is a gift we often take for granted, but when faced with the possibility of losing one's vision, it can be devastating. When my name was called I was still confident this would be my first and last visit. After hours of exams, eye drops, ultra-sounds and tests I never imagined existed, my new physician, Doctor Jose Pulido delivered the life changing diagnosis that I had a rare (one in one million) intra-ocular melanoma. After hearing the word melanoma, I must confess I experienced a numbing shock that stayed with me until we were entering the elevator to the parking ramp to return home. The reality that I had a fast growing tumor normally considered a dangerous skin cancer inside my eye was unthinkable.

I was scheduled to return to the clinic on my sixty-fourth birthday for more tests, including a CT scan that would reveal if the cancer had spread to the liver or lungs, the most vulnerable areas of the body for this form of cancer. On December 10, 2007, I underwent radioactive plaque surgery where the muscles of my left eye were cut and a small brass disc was inserted, and placed at the back of the wall of my eye behind the tumor. The disc resembled a bottle cap and contained tiny seeds of radioactive iodine. The muscles were re-sutured and the disc remained in place for four days when it was finally removed. I went home to Owatonna with a metal protective cover over my extremely painful eye and with renewed hope that the tumor would shrink and eventually die.

My recovery was considered normal and the tumor appeared to be shrinking. After months of attempting to adapt to double vision, lack of depth perception, and dizziness, I gradually regained most of my vision. Sometime during my ensuing treatments, I was informed that my newest scan showed suspicious spots on my lungs that eventually were not considered cancerous but would have to be monitored. It was at this time in my very busy life that I was forced to face the reality that I could die. I had to give my complete attention and focus on what I really believed in with my heart and soul. I struggled with guilt wondering what would happen to my family if I did not survive, and what the real priorities were if my time here on earth was limited. I was forced to examine who or what God was, and that alone was a remarkably revealing spiritual journey, because my faith or religion was one area I had never questioned. I began to realize I looked at people differently and was much more accepting of what I considered to be their shortcomings. I found new heroes everywhere and I also realized how much my husband and six children loved me. Last of all, I finished and published the novel I had been struggling with for years. My first novel, *Forgive Me Father* is now a reality, and I am proud to say I have almost completed the sequel.

In July of 2008, my confrontation with my new dark companion took another unexpected turn when I experienced hemorrhaging in the affected eye and loss of vision. This was considered breakthrough bleeding caused by the tumor dying. In an attempt to restore my vision in April of 2009, I underwent a vitrectomy to remove the cloudy fluid that contained unabsorbed blood. Later, it was discovered I had developed a cataract, a common side effect of the radiation and had surgery in June of 2009 to remove it. The surgery was successful but I soon experienced more bleeding and vision loss. This was followed by eight or nine injections of the drug Avastin directly into my eye in an attempt to control the bleeding. A new diagnosis in October revealed signs of possible radiation retinopathy or damage to the retina from the exposure of radiation during the initial surgery. In April of 2011, I was advised to continue with the eye injections but I declined. The vision in my left eye has improved but remains limited, similar to what one might experience if Vaseline was smeared on the lens of one's glasses.

Several months ago I read a remarkable book, *The Mind's Eye,* by Oliver Sacks, a medical doctor who experienced an intra-ocular melanoma in his right eye. In his concise clinical analysis of his experience, he examines the possibility that when one sense is diminished or taken away there may be evidence that in unique cases, the mind, or brain may compensate for the loss. This insight wakened in me that my dark confrontation with unexpected illness did not come without its own reward. I now see and perceive the world differently and am acutely aware that each day is a blessing, not to be squandered. My initial loss of sight had become a window of valuable insights. To quote Henry Miller, *"One's destination is never a place, but rather a new way of looking at things".* My gift in return for coming to terms with my dark companion is to educate others about this rare condition, and the importance of regular eye exams.

TEARS

Paul H. Waytz, M.D.

I am a rheumatologist, a physician subspecializing in diseases that primarily affect the musculoskeletal system, especially the joints. The overwhelming majority of people we see have chronic illnesses because of unknown disturbances of the immune system. Patients experience pain, stiffness, and weakness, among other symptoms. They have the potential for significant joint damage, loss of mobility, disability, and problems with the simple, everyday tasks most of us take for granted. Contrary to popular belief, complaints usually start between the ages of twenty and forty. Each patient is unique in how they are affected as well as how they affect those around them.

Judy once called me long distance from Florida. She quickly grew annoyed when I could not tell her what her rash was simply from her description over the telephone. On a different occasion, she called me and became annoyed when I couldn't tell her exactly why she was having so much pain in her knee two weeks after she fractured the lower portion of her thighbone. Then, about a year ago, she called me and, once again, voiced an annoyed tone when I could not tell her if she should or should not baby-sit her two-year old granddaughter who may or may not have been exposed to strep at a birthday party.

Recently, it was a normal day—whatever normal means after thirty years in private practice—and Judy was in for her regular follow-up visit. She is fifty-five and no longer working; I have known her more than ten years. She has primary Sjogren's syndrome with mild, associated arthritis. Sjogren's syndrome is an autoimmune disease of unknown cause characterized primarily by extreme dryness of the mouth and eyes because of damage to saliva and tear glands. From the time Judy started medication, she has never had any symptoms or signs indicating that things were progressing or transforming to some more ominous problem, notwithstanding that the disease itself is serious enough.

On this day, as things were winding down with her appointment, Judy reviewed with me that she had had a difficult year emotionally: her father died, one of her children had a premature baby, she was now being required to handle a number of family matters that she did not feel prepared to do. She told me that her physical health was holding well, but she was experiencing a particular difficulty: she couldn't make tears. She could no longer cry. As hard as she worked at it, and for all of the right reasons, she just could not weep. She understood that it was because of her Sjogren's syndrome, but this admission implied more, both to me and to her.

We all understand that crying is a basic human emotional response. Of all people, I should know. I cried when my favorite baseball team won the World Series. I so often well up when hearing of charitable good deeds or seeing unexpected sweetness in the news, my family and friends come to expect it and are no longer embarrassed on my behalf.

But, what if I could not cry; what if I were physically unable? After expressing my empathy toward Judy, I walked out of my ordinary examination room feeling a suddenly rooted need for some personal examination.

Within just minutes, previously considered, but recurring elemental thoughts went through my head: "Why did I choose this profession and subspecialty?" "What do we give?" and even the existential and truly trite "What am I actually doing here?"

What gifts we embrace and utilize—the patience to listen, the ability to feel (both physically and internally), and the skill to formulate a plan—-often remain a mystery to me. Giving so often implies a transferring, a bestowing, from one person to another. We all go through our days as actors, quickly and necessarily changing roles in the very appropriate service of those seeking our professional care and advice. But along the way, we sometimes have to stop and ask ourselves: Do we truly meet needs of patients more often than not? Do we justify the fact that they are actually paying us? In Judy's case, was the fact that all I could offer her was empathy a good and decent enough response?

Not to be lost, too, is the question of how these patients change us and affect our own needs. Do we let ourselves realize how lucky we are to be serving others, and, therefore, ourselves as well?

It all circles back to compassion, but compassion is both an insufficient word and feeling. We cannot assume it nor is it somehow foisted upon us. The question I repeatedly ask myself is: How far does compassion extend and is there a limit? We interact with strangers who, if anything, are not strange at all. What does the next person want: Does a poor person want money, does a sad person want a joke or consolation? We give drugs, time, solace, and experience utilizing varying and always-evolving degrees of rationale, reasonableness, and responsibility. Will an innocent (or not so innocent) remark by a patient set off another chain of questions and introspection? Can we give these notions due time and respect? And then we have to make sure we appear presentable enough for the next patient and move on.

During free-floating and free-associating moments, I pester myself with questions like these that may or may not be answerable. In that vein, I often consider rheumatology a perfect metaphor. We deal with basic components of the human condition including pain, stiffness, loss of mobility, weakness, and depression. As someone who prefers to read fiction, I can easily get lost in all of these facets. I find myself wondering what people are doing when they walk out of my office and through the door of their own homes and workplaces to interact with families and their unique world. Will they do what is told and suggested and, if so, will they respond medically? Life would be different, perhaps even simpler, if rheumatology were more black and white and more predictable. There might be less chaos and change for patients and doctors. But surely there wouldn't be the challenge. And there certainly would be far fewer of these short stories.

I think I need to cry for Judy. I have convinced myself that that is my burden. If it's not my professional burden, it is my burden as a fellow human being. Collectively, do we all need to weep for Judy and everyone who cannot shed their own tears no matter the reason? These are universal questions of how much we ask for as well as how we explore the lines where professionalism and humanity intersect. We all have jobs to do, but how do we best fulfill those responsibilities and also best foster a necessary and truly human collusion of spirit?

MIMI MAY I?

Sandra Frederiksen Weicht

Two precious grandbabies sit in front of me. Carlee is four and Matthew, one.

A few minutes ago, they bound through the front door like tightly wound springs breaking loose. I grab a pillow and hold it to my chest. Carlee runs up, stops within a foot of me, and states, "Mommy said we cannot run at you because of your owie."

Kid-size wrought iron chairs are in front of my recliner; the bundles of energy perch on or more accurately hover over them. Excitedly, they chatter, "You were in the hospital. The doctors cut out the cancer. You have bad owies on your boobies. We can't run into you or it will hurt. You can't pick us up for a long time." Joy and love push out fear and uncertainty on my emotional roller coaster.

Can it only be a month ago? January tenth, you never forget the day of discovery. My reflection in the bathroom mirror wasn't right. A raised area surrounded the nipple on my left breast. The nipple wasn't in the middle of the areole. Staring at the woman in the mirror, I knew in my heart of hearts what it meant. I called my hubby and asked if he'd noticed any irregularities. He hadn't.

Monday, the twelfth, my gynecologist fit me in early. She scheduled a mammogram and ultra sound at the Breast Center. There was a cancelation. The next open appointment was ten days away. Coincidence? No. God was already holding me.

Wednesday we went back to the Breast Center for a core biopsy. The doctor confirmed it was cancer. I cannot remember any of that conversation. When a nurse came in, I questioned why my husband wasn't brought in before the doctor talked to me. The nurse went over more information; John was still in the waiting room, not by my side. In the fog of those moments I remember whispering to him, "It is breast cancer!" Later, I learned it was infiltrating lobular carcinoma, nine centimeters in size.

There was no time to absorb the diagnosis. That night I sent a short email to immediate family and a few close friends asking for prayers.

Friday, the sixteenth was a surgeon consult. John and a dear friend were with me. Both were invaluable. Extra ears and the medical knowledge, my friend had helped get answers to questions I didn't even know to ask.

The whirlwind kept spiraling. Monday, one week after discovery, was another trip to the Breast Center for more tests. The MRI showed a mass in the left breast and a small area in the right breast.

It was time to call in our arsenal. An email was sent to family and friends. Prayers and support were needed as never before. They showered us with both. We requested no phone calls. Repeating it over and over was too hard. Emails, cards, and promises of prayers and help poured in.

The next week the surgeons explained tests and the process of the mastectomy and reconstruction. It was my choice to have a bilateral or double mastectomy. The lessened chance of reoccurrence and the even physical appearance were important to me. I needed to know how fast all of this had to happen. Two important events were imminent. It could wait weeks but not months.

The next week, we watched Carlee and Matthew while their folks were on vacation. Exhaustion claimed John and I each night from caring for those bundles of energy after daycare until they were in their beds recharging for the next day.

At the end of January, our fourth grandbaby was due. How exciting! Our daughter, son-in-law, and third grandchild, Randall, were in their new home. It was a two and a half hour drive. We would go up Friday, January 30th, and I'd stay for a week. My daughter was under so much stress her doctor induced her. That evening our precious Tanner entered our lives. We were now blessed with four beautiful, healthy grandbabies. John returned the next weekend and brought me home to our new reality and more doctors' appointments.

We met my oncologist on February 5th. It was important she was the right doctor for me. She would be the main player in my immediate future. She was wonderful. We clicked.

February 11th arrived; we met the surgeons at the hospital. After final consults, they did their "art work" on me. It was time for surgery. John, our son and wife, three very close friends, and our pastor were there. While our pastor was praying, our beautiful daughter-in-law softly wept. I hugged her and told her it would be okay no matter where I woke up.

After surgery, expanders were where the implants would go. I didn't lose my shape and was never without my breasts. They were different, but my chest wasn't flat.

Between family and friends visiting and the hubbub of hospital life, time flew. We were sent home to figure out our new life.

Now there are a couple sweet little ones asking, "Mimi, may I come up to you? Mimi, may I sit on your lap? Mimi, may I hug you? Mimi, I love you."

A few weeks later, precocious Carlee walked in on me while I was dressing. She didn't bat an eye. She saw my "new" breasts and declared, "Oh, Mimi, you have scratches!" They were my scars. No trauma to that one. She accepted everything.

Because of the double mastectomy; no radiation was required and only four chemo treatments, one every twenty-one days. It took lots of work, and one round of chemo was administrated while on vacation in Florida.

Looking back, my side effects were minimal. They was the usual weight gain, queasy tummy, skin—especially the torso—very sensitive, constipation, diarrhea that caused a sore bottom, thrush, food tasting odd, rashes, fatigue, scalp acne that looked like little bug bites, night sweats, and achy fingers, toes, and nails. Medications kept them in check. It was a blessing to have had an easier ordeal than most. I felt guilty, many get deathly ill.

My hair was a main defining factor. April first, how fitting April Fools Day, in the shower my hands became covered with hair! I called my dear friend and asked her to cut off my hair. Having it fall out would be horrid. She and I got through it with tears and a huge bottle of wine. My head resembled a "very old" Grandpa's head. The stubble looked awful. Scarves and skullcaps covered the poor thing for six months.

The beginning of January 2009 was one of the most frightening times of my life. My husband, family and friends' prayers and support buoyed me up. The most important lesson I learned was no matter what I will ever go through, God surrounds me with His angels' wings.

I am blessed.

My husband was diagnosed with esophageal cancer exactly one year after my breast cancer diagnosis. This poem was written last Christmas to celebrate our two and three years survival and sweet precious extra life together.

CHRISTMAS

Cancer

Horrible

Ravishing

Invasive

Surrender

T*ears*

Miracles

Angel Wings

Savior

RACHEL D. NEMITZ

It was my death sentence.

The surgeon told me I had breast cancer, and I had never known a survivor. He said it was infiltrating ductal carcinoma and infiltrating lobular carcinoma—a large stage two. I only heard, "You have a large breast cancer." Having had previous biopsies, I was not worried and expected this would be just another benign lump. Later, reading the surgeon's notes he had written, "She showed no emotion and asked no questions, an unusual reaction."

In seventeen years, I had never skipped my annual checkup with the usual Pap smear and mammogram. But the year I turned sixty-two, retired and relocated, I didn't take the time to find a new doctor and have a physical. The next year, I did visit an OB/GYN. After the examination, he walked me down the hall for a mammogram and then scheduled me to see a surgeon the next day and the following day I had a biopsy. The surgeon sat beside me and told me I had breast cancer. A week later, a lumpectomy was performed and lymph nodes removed.

I lived with my daughter, Dawn, and her husband, Kip. When I arrived home from the doctor's office, Dawn was at work but Kip was there and asked me what the doctor had said.

"No shit?" he asked.

"No shit," I answered and went downstairs to my little apartment. I sat at the computer, with tears running down my face, and pulled up Scrabble as doom-filled scenes ran through my head. I was afraid. Not so much of death but afraid I might not have the courage needed to face what was ahead of me. I was sitting there, the tears flowing, when Dawn walked in. I don't remember our conversation but she went to the library and brought back several recently published books on breast cancer.

The next morning I drove to my lakeside cabin, the books lying on the seat beside me. I read, cried, threw things and made a list of questions; then I called the surgeon's oncology nurse. She and I talked for over an hour. Unhurried, she answered all my questions. I stopped crying. My fight began.

A MUGA test revealed my heart would not withstand the preferred chemotherapy. As a result, instead of having four sessions of intravenous chemo I had two intravenous sessions a month for six months and took pills for two weeks each month. Because of the weaker chemotherapy and taking pills, rather than having that particular drug go directly into the bloodstream, I never lost my hair. Hallelujah! My family insisted one of them accompany me to every chemo and radiation session although I certainly could have gone alone.

After my first chemotherapy, I felt okay—just a little weird. Dawn and I drove to see Kim, my oldest daughter, there the three of us celebrated with champagne. Thanks to the nausea drug, Zofran (Compazine didn't do the job) only once did I experience that horrible nausea that makes you pray for death to come quickly. During this time, we discovered a lump in my left breast that turned out to be lobular carcinoma in situ, meaning it was encapsulated and had not spread. We continued with the original treatment plan.

Three months into chemotherapy, I became agitated, even frenetic. I couldn't set still and moved from one chair to another, to the bed, to the couch, and even out into winter's cold blast. I could not settle down enough to sleep, watch television or read. I was convinced I had gone crazy. The oncologist refused to help me saying he'd never heard of such a thing. I called my general practitioner and asked to be referred to a psychiatrist. "Come see me right away," he said.

Sleeping pills helped but the problem was my thyroid. Twenty years previously, a malignancy had been removed from my thyroid. What remained was being affected by the chemotherapy. My wonderful kind, gentle and caring surgeon removed the remaining thyroid. He explained that it might be difficult to locate the vocal cords because of scar tissue from the earlier surgery, and reassuringly, he said, "You pay me a lot of money to make sure you can still talk after I'm through."

Nevertheless, it was scary.

I'd almost finished the thirty-three radiation treatments but my mind was fuzzy...like a head full of cotton balls. Instead of stepping down onto the balcony to watch the grandkids play basketball, I stepped out and fell breaking both bones in my lower right leg. As my leg broke, I saw in my mind a jagged white line that looked exactly like the break shown on the x-ray. Six weeks in a cast.

Chemo and radiation were over. The leg healed. I had a full head of hair. My mind was clearer. Since my cancer grew off hormones, the oncologist insisted I take Tamoxifen. After reading everything I could find on Tamoxifen, I was reluctant. There were many possible side effects and one could never know if it had worked. After debating for a couple of months, I decided the doctor should know best and began the five-year protocol.

A couple of years later, my sister, Eltrie, was diagnosed with breast cancer. She elected to have her breast removed and undergo radiation but not chemotherapy or hormone therapy. I went to Arkansas to be with her as she recuperated and to work with Social Services and arrange for someone to help her. I hated the long, ugly scar left on her chest. Eltrie lived another two years.

Returning home, it was time for my checkup. A lobular carcinoma in situ was found in the breast that had undergone radiation. The surgeon, general practitioner and the oncologist, all told me, "Get rid of those things or they'll kill you." So, I had a double mastectomy.

Remembering Eltrie's large, ugly scar I thought I'd like to have reconstruction. I discussed this with a counselor who told me she could never be so narcissistic. Her husband would love her just as much without her breasts. I was offended. My husband was dead; I had no lover and certainly didn't think I was narcissistic. So much for her counseling. I researched the different types of reconstruction and opted for the one where the surgeon brings fat and a blood supply from the abdomen up under the skin to construct a new breast. After consulting two plastic surgeons, I was told that, because of a scar from my gall bladder operation, the procedure would involve a micro surgeon (if I could find one who would do it) and I would be taking a greater risk. I decided on saline implants. The surgery went smoothly, pain was minimal and I never felt like I had lost my breasts.

Eleven years have passed. My life has been full and satisfying. I now know many survivors. Several of them are my friends. They are brave, loving people with a deep understanding of human nature and a great appreciation for all life.

ROAD TO HOPE

Paula Nelson-Guenther

"Time for pie," I announced to the male contingency who had sneaked to the den for the Dallas versus Seattle football game, avoiding clean-up duty. "We have apple, pumpkin and pecan. Who wants what? Erick? Todd? Joe?"

Joe! JOE! WHAT'S WRONG?" Slumped in the huge leather chair, his head tilted back as the eyes, lips and jaw drooped, the entire right side of the body unmovable.

"Quick, call 911!" someone yelled. "Looks like a stroke."

Holidays. Some are electric, exciting and exhilarating; others dreadfully boring. Thanksgiving 2008 was none of these. It was catastrophic.

Fortunately, we were ten minutes from one of the leading stroke centers in the Minneapolis/St. Paul area, United Hospital, where the medicine t-PA (Tissue Plasminogen Activator) was administered within the three-hour time requirement.

"Shalom," the intensive care nurse spoke, gently placing a warm hand on my arm. "You may see your husband now." Sensitive comment, I thought, standing immobile in the emergency unit at the St. Paul hospital while several personnel hustled about, one by one thrusting unsigned paperwork in my hand.

A blur of activity dominated the next forty-eight hours. Joe's right side remained paralyzed, the result of major injury to the left carotid artery, which also affected the communication center of the brain's left hemisphere, the Broca area. Damage was massive leaving him unable to talk, read or write although he understood spoken language.

Joe had no known risk factors, making the stroke a shock to everyone who knew him. In addition, he had years of healthy eating, while keeping a proper weight and an active lifestyle.

In-patient physical, occupational and speech therapy began a few days later. The grueling three-hour a day, six day a week rehabilitation continued for a month. I arrived at the hospital early in the morning, staying until late afternoon recording almost all of Joe's sessions: strapped to the treadmill walking, practicing on the balance beam, tossing rubber balls into nets; and flexing the fingers stacking blocks, counting coins and dialing telephone numbers.

"Okay, Joe, you've done great!" exclaimed the young energetic therapist. "Today we're going to do the Wii game. How about ski racing? We'll use the Balance Beam."

Questions to Joe's physicians and therapists about his future prognosis, however, were always met with hesitant, masked faces. "We really can't tell at this point," said one. Another cautioned, "Progress is so individual." A third offered formulas for tracking the progression of stroke survivors, but a fourth said this was now outdated. Not very optimistic, nor encouraging.

Physically Joe did well, gradually gaining the use of his legs, arms and other bodily functions. Balance developed too. Problems continued, however, with speaking, reading, writing and swallowing. Progress in these areas seemed bleak, and I wondered how long complete healing would take.

December twenty-four, Joe was discharged and we drove home to Duluth, Minnesota to an empty, cold house. For the first time ever, we postponed holiday celebrations as both of us were exhausted and distressed with such a heavy burden suddenly added to our lives.

My new role as a 24/7 caregiver began.

Friends and family's reactions shocked me. Some completely dropped out of our lives, two callously informing me of their decisions. A family member expounded, "I'm not going to take care of another baby," referring to my husband. Others were especially caring and kind, unexpectedly volunteering to help in numerous ways. Outside of relatives and friends, the kindest of all were waiters and salespeople who patiently tolerated Joe's gestures and gyrations as he struggled with communication.

Treatment continued in Duluth. Joe exceeded expectations physically and the ability to once again ballroom dance and downhill ski became the Winter 2009 goal. "Happy February14th birthday, sweetheart," I whispered as we danced familiar waltzes, swings, tangos, rumbas, fox trots and polkas. He remembered all of the steps! We were ecstatic!

Two weeks later he snow skied. "You've done the Bunny Hill just fine," confirmed his special needs teacher. "Now you're ready for the Big Hills. Go for it!" We spent the entire next day skiing. Life was looking up. However, although he could ski and swallow, he still was unable to talk, read or write.

Just as Joe's health improved, mine started failing. How could this be as I had always been healthy? April, diet and exercise no longer controlled my diabetes and I needed more treatment. In addition, my cholesterol numbers were exceptionally high. Soon medicine controlled my being.

That same month, Joe had his first seizure, leaving him unconscious. Nine more seizures interrupted Joe's progress by slowing his physical and mental growth. Finally, a workable medical protocol regulated the sudden attacks.

April continued as our worst month. Another major shock surfaced as my yearly physical exam showed a dangerously blocked aortic valve along with an obstructed coronary artery. Where were the warning signs? The minor heart murmur discovered a few years ago?

I visited the surgeon. "The good news is that you're in excellent health for your age and the heart is not damaged yet."

"But what about...?" I began, hoping to ask about my care giving responsibilities.

"You'll pop right back. We'll use a mechanical valve researched right here in Minnesota by Medtronic." I wondered, but scheduled the open-heart surgery in July.

The physician was correct as my good health quickly returned; but consequently, more medicine and dietary restrictions dominated my life.

Worries mounted as neither Joe nor I could drive for six weeks. Another burden seemed insurmountable. Still, as with the other concerns, these too evolved.

Summer faded into Fall and Joe's speech therapy continued. We also began music therapy. As a musician, I reinforced Joe's speech drills through exercises, rhythms songs. Joe surprised the family December 2010 by singing *"Silent Night,"* and six other pieces with most of the words clearly understandable. Everyone was speechless.

Winter 2010, both of us plunged into a deep gloom precipitated by disappointment and impatience. I was intent at keeping Joe positive and upbeat; he was frustrated because of the diligent speech and music exercises although he now could speak ten words.

So, together we made a "back-to-health" plan. First, we started a rigorous program of walking, skiing, and aerobic exercise. Next, we consciously associated with upbeat people.

"Should we see *How to Talk Minnesotan* again?" I asked. "Felt great to laugh two hours straight!"

"Yes," Joe answered, using one of his new words. Enjoying comedy in theaters, movies, television shows; and simply laughing, making light of our serious situation, was another point in our pact.

We increased our activity in church, clubs and other organizations, volunteering in special interest activities and projects. We continued our healthy eating plan.

Living is easier now. Adjustments continue, however, particularly with Joe's complex "relearning" personality. He is as a three-year-old starting to talk, a six-year-old learning to read and write, and a teenager working at making wise decisions, all rolled into one seventy-three-year-old.

Our misfortunes seem minor now; we know and appreciate what is possible. Margaret Mitchell, in the final line of *Gone With The Wind* wrote, "After all, tomorrow is another day."

Yes, life does go on.

MY MOTHER'S STORY

Amy Lindgren

I look at my face in the mirror for the hundredth time—it isn't my face anymore, it's my mother's. Two years older than she was at her death, I have finally become her entirely—or the her she would have been. This is what she would have looked like healthy. Only she was rarely healthy, in my memory at least.

Her illness arrived before I was born, at least parts of it. The mental illness must have been there, lying in wait, or how else could it have bloomed so fully? Perhaps the cancers were waiting too, encoded in her DNA. Perhaps they're waiting in my DNA as well? All my life I have imagined dying young from a disease, if only because that was the plan I understood best. If the children of teachers become teachers, and doctors beget doctors, wouldn't I also inherit my mother's occupation, which seemed to be illness?

So I have been waiting for illness all my life, never quite trusting my health. Once when I found a lump in my breast, I felt both fear and vindication. You're late, I said out loud. I expected you years ago. But it was a false alarm and I'm still waiting.

My mother didn't have to wait. The first cancer appeared when I was five and she was thirty-one. That one should have killed her. Cervical cancer in the 1960s was nothing to play with. Later, when a fellow waitress at the supper club was diagnosed with the same disease, she told my mother, I'm not worried; you're my role model and you survived. Of course the friend died. My mother felt guilty for years.

When did she begin shutting herself in the bedroom? I can't remember a time when my mother didn't retreat that way. I do remember hours alone on the braided rug in our rambler, playing with Lincoln logs and stuffed animals, whiling away the hours. I wasn't school age yet, but I was very self-sufficient. When I was finally four, my mother convinced the school to take me a year early, then walked me the five blocks to the school door. I walked alone every day thereafter, in all weather, amazed to learn later that some kids got rides when it was sleeting. It wasn't a bad childhood in that way—just lonely.

Does this sound like a needy adult, looking back with grief on a lost childhood? Most days I don't feel that way. In truth, I'm amazed to be here at all, and not just because I imagine an illness that is late in arriving. We understand now what post-partum depression can do, particularly if it isn't treated. My mother was taken away for a while after my birth when she was found throttling my older sister. I learned this as an adult but I never doubted the story. I had seen the quick flash when my mother's temper was about to let go, and had witnessed the brutality when it did. I had even felt her hands at my own throat once, and watched her eyes widen in recognition at what she was doing before she loosened her grip. That was an incident we never talked about. If my father had known, there would have been trouble.

When my mother finally died at age forty-seven, of the second or third cancer— there's been some confusion in our memories about skin cancers in her thirties—when she died, I knew that she would have rather lived. Not just because the last cancer was a beast, as lung cancer can be. But because she was finally, finally, grasping the reins on her own life. A divorce at thirty-six, her GED at forty, exploring new careers at forty-one. And even a trip to rehab at forty-six. What irony that the illness she wasn't expecting arrived just as she was vanquishing the one she had known all her adult life. The day she was to be released from alcohol treatment, her Big Book and well wishes in hand, the biopsy came back positive. Orderlies arrived in the rehab wing of the hospital to load her things onto a gurney bound for the surgical wing. The next day, when she should have been starting a new life of AA meetings and job search, she was moaning in pain from having her lung removed.

The ten months that followed were nightmarish and surreal. I had always known it would end this way, if only because I lacked the imagination to expect otherwise. At nineteen, I had always lived with her illness as my dark companion. My sister had the sense to run away into the juvenile justice system. Her way of growing up was ten times more difficult but she was spared the daily ups and downs of progressive illness. Unburdened by lessons in cleaning surgical wounds and suctioning trachs, she was able to maintain a distance.

Even with all that, I miss my mom.

I write the alternate lives in my mind. If her illness was a dark companion while she lived, her hypothetical health is my bright companion now. Seeing her face in the mirror when I brush my teeth, I can't help musing. What if she had come from rehab into a new world of supportive AA friends and a job she loved—perhaps arranging flowers and growing plants? What if she had stayed sober and we got to spend afternoons shopping? What if I could take her somewhere amazing, like Mexico or Brazil? What if she had met my husband? I know she would have loved him.

She would have been seventy-seven last Christmas and Easter will mark the thirtieth anniversary of her death. The irony of giving two holidays over to these remembrances isn't lost on me. The celebrations we didn't mark in her lifetime are filled with her presence now.

She lives somewhere now, but I don't know where. When she died, my sister and I were sleeping in her hospital room, folded into vinyl chairs by the bed. At four AM., Nancy heard mom's breathing change, and she nudged me awake. We held hands in a chain, my sister linking my mother and me, as mom took her last breath. I was exhausted, numb, not thinking clearly. And yet, I have never disbelieved the image that flew, unbidden, into my tired mind as my mother left this earth: At once, I saw her as a young woman, a bouquet of bright balloons rising from an uplifted arm as she ran joyfully across a grassy hilltop in the sunshine. I saw my mother as clearly as in a movie, free and happy and out of the darkness of her illnesses. And even though I never knew her that way, somehow I recognized that young, free woman as her real self. I'm grateful for the image; it's the way I choose to remember her.

BONNIE GINTIS

When I took the oath as a physician on graduation day from Osteopathic medical school in 1986, I promised to listen deeply, to feel the messages conveyed by my patients' bodies, especially their bones, not knowing what that promise would eventually entail. After years of caring for people and devoting my studies and perceptual training to receiving the stories of other people's bones, my own bones call out more loudly than anything I've ever heard. My bones have become passageways for breast cancer to spread its cryptic message. I promised to listen, and now I hear an unexpected language spoken in a strange tempo that sounds like the static blur of a shortwave radio transmitting a distress signal from a far away place in the night.

I yearn to understand the language of bones, of the dialect spoken by the cancer in my bones. What is the grammar of cancer? With what does its rhythm and cadence synchronize? A tumor bulges from within my sternum, hovering over my beating heart. Is there communication between my heart and the tumor, or is cancer like a sociopath, wreaking havoc and causing harm without empathy for the suffering it causes? The paradox is that this cancer in my bones is essentially made from my own cells. Do I have cancer, or does it have me? Is it mine? Can it be had? Is it an "it," or is it me? Have I been inflicted or gifted by this growing presence within me?

When I can't understand something, I turn towards the sensation of my moving breath, and look for resemblances and resonances with water. I lay in bed late at night when I cannot sleep and ride the fluid breath inside my bones.

When I take this ride, I clearly see that the common feeling many of us have, that our bones are solid, is an illusion. The average bone is about twenty percent water. What an interesting way for the body to store and utilize water! Water is somewhat useless without a functional container. If you carried water in a plastic bag, it would not be handy when you got thirsty. If you stored your drinking water inside your car's tires, you would have no access to it when you needed a drink. The human body is an incredibly functional container for its seventy percent water content; its spaces, cells, and tissues form the vessel for its fluid-based form. Some mysterious set of codes and signals organizes our amorphous sac-of-water bodies into a highly functional form, and in my case, these signals have been distorted allowing cancer to overgrow inside my bones.

I oscillate from sensation to science, from memoir to philosophy every time I hit a cancerous bump in the road. I try to breathe and just let it be, but I become distracted by the dissonance between what I think about the body and what mine is actually doing.

Listening to the distress signals emanating from my bones, I am reminded of my promise. Bones carry promises from one point in time to another. The mineral and fluid matrix resonates and receives signals simultaneously from the past and future. Life unfolds from all directions, not necessarily in a linear progression, into all directions through our bones. My bones will bridge the past and future assimilating food and water, the wake of desire and longing, the residues of repetition and impact, and the hardened reactions to shock and trauma. The messages of my bones will persist whether buried or burned. The call of the shadow arises from deep in the marrow. A light cannot shine in such an enclosed space, but a river can flow in the darkness. A message arises from the darkness and I hear it emerge as a ripple in the stream of my consciousness. As I adapt to the dark, I hear a distant Voice, whispering, calling out an as yet unimagined message about allowing the next moment of my life to flow into the present. The response to this call, to such profound loss, is nothing short of radical re-imagination. I promised to listen.

OUT OF DARKNESS

Kirsten Young

Life radically changed for me January 9, 2007, when exploratory surgery to remove a grapefruit-sized cyst on my right ovary revealed metastatic ovarian cancer. The surgeons made an incision from above my navel to the pubic bone to remove the cancerous ovaries, fallopian tubes, a part of the momentum, and lesions on the peritoneum (the lining of the abdominal cavity). When I awoke in recovery, my husband told me the frightening findings. Two weeks earlier, my gynecologist had suggested the cyst may be cancerous and I told my Associate Director at Morrison County Public Health. She looked somber as she cautioned, "If so, you're in for the fight of your life."

On Monday, January 8, the Department's annual all-staff retreat went on as planned, but I stayed at the office to tie up as many loose ends as possible. I joined the group for lunch and to tell my staff about the scheduled surgery. Throughout the day, I had recurring thoughts that this might be my last day on the job for a while or even my last workday ever.

My two children arrived at the hospital in early evening stricken with fear. They could not fathom how their mother with such a healthy lifestyle could now have late stage cancer. Despite my stoic nature, I felt shaken by this grave diagnosis. Life had turned dark.

The next morning, the oncologist assigned my case arrived. He was brief. "You have serous adenocarcinoma, Stage III-C. It's not curable, but it is treatable and we will use the gold standard, cisplatin and taxol, to treat it." He explained the six cycles of treatment: hospitalization for twenty-four hour intravenous chemo followed by an intraperitoneal infusion to bathe the abdominal cavity in another chemical for four hours. Eight days after the IV infusion, I would receive another intraperitoneal infusion at the Coborn Cancer Center. He finished with these words: "This cancer will recur. When it does, we'll treat it again. It's like a chronic disease."

Now I felt even more overwhelmed and cheated. I started receiving flowers and visitors, but I had few words for these dear people who obviously cared about me. Cardiac problems were a familiar scourge in my family, not cancer. An oncology nurse from the Cancer Center visited and I learned the chemotherapy would begin in early February after two infusion ports were surgically inserted at the hospital, one below the right collarbone and the other below the lowest right rib. I'd be the Center's second ovarian cancer patient treated this way.

During the hospitalization, I roamed the halls. Other than the surgical pain, I felt physically well but continued to be incredulous that millions of cancer cells had been silently growing in my innards. Obviously, my body was trying to get my attention; my life was out of balance and the cancer had developed due to a variety of reasons. My body had been saying "no" via various maladies I experienced over the previous three years—four orthopedic surgeries, a detached retina, and a major heart attack. I knew I needed to quit my rewarding job. As I learned about survival statistics for late stage ovarian cancer, I anticipated a shorter lifespan and wanted to spend it with family.

The financial ramifications of retiring were worrisome. When my husband left our home in Little Falls in April to live at his lake home fifty miles away, we put our house up for sale. I bought a home in Sauk Rapids for my daughter, her four year old son, Brock, and me, took on a sizable mortgage and moved in September. Before my 63rd birthday on April thirteen, my planned job termination date, my eligibility for disability was confirmed. I would be able to pay my bills. Nevertheless, it was disconcerting to know that I qualified based on my projected short lifespan. The oncologist's medical report stated my disability was permanent and my prognosis guarded. I knew this, but it still was chilling to see it in print.

Reading numerous books about cancer expanded my knowledge and perspective. I became convinced that a holistic approach would bring harmony to mind, body and spirit—critical to my healing. To the chemotherapy I added alternative therapies—walking, eating nutritious foods, visualization, acupuncture, massage, yoga, singing and journaling. I had engaged in each of these alternative therapies at various times, but never in concert.

Occasional trips to Little Falls to see friends helped. Because Brock's mom was gone for twelve hours each day with a long commute to her job in Brooklyn Center, I was his primary caregiver. Taking him to preschool, shopping, meal preparation, laundry, and household chores gave me purpose.

Severe depletion of white and red blood cells required injections after each chemo session to boost their numbers. Other side effects included bowel problems, bloody nasal discharge, poor appetite, hair loss, nausea, neuropathy, fatigue and sleeplessness. With each chemo session, the effects grew worse to the point that I wanted to quit after the fifth session and wrote in my journal, *Stop the chemo now*! When I shared this with the acupuncturist, he urged me to continue and emphasized, "Finishing might make all the difference."

After each chemotherapy treatment, I had excessive urination to remove the chemicals and fluids from my body. Brock had to avoid using our usually shared bathroom because of the toxicity from the urine spray into the toilet. He also had to be reminded not to bump me when I had a needle in the top port prior to a chemo session.

Despite the adversities, many good things eased my way during this challenging time. I completed the chemotherapy, experienced excellent care from health care providers, and benefitted from the prayers and support of colleagues at work, family, church members and friends. Public Health friends sent a photo that showed their right hands grouped together, each wearing a cancer bracelet.

I valued my good health insurance. Moving to Sauk Rapids meant a drive of only four miles to the hospital and cancer center where I spent so much time for seven months. After completion of the chemotherapy regimen, I received two units of stacked red blood cells. This brought color back to my face and relieved the fatigue. A CT scan confirmed cancer remission. Light was returning.

Because my usual exuberance for life had been severely taxed, I sought help from a psychologist I knew in Little Falls. I relayed my fear that I would not see Brock grow up. She reminded me of resilience I had shown during other difficult times and suggested that I write my life story as a legacy for him. This idea was captivating and I began a memoir, took writing classes and joined a writer's group. I learned to find joy in the present and began to live more simply and mindfully. In September, 2007, I began serving on a newly formed Cancer Survivorship Advisory Council at the Cancer Center to provide ideas for programming.

On January 9, 2012, five years after my devastating diagnosis, a CT scan and blood tests show I continue to be cancer-free. I am fortunate, indeed!

THE POWER OF PRAYER

Joy Fisher

The movie had ended, but I could not lift myself from the seat. The room whirled around me blurring the dimensions and blending the colors. I tried to force my eyes to focus on the seat in front of me but it was as if I were looking through a fishbowl of water, my eyes never quite able to clear. I blinked hard and tried to shake my head, but that brought on a wave of nausea so forceful I covered my mouth and inhaled deeply through my nose. The back of my head was pulling me downward to the floor; tiny droplets of sweat were forming on my brow and running down my face and neck in narrow rivers. I was upright now and plastered against the fuzzy carpet of the theater walls hanging on to the longest threads that my fingers could grasp. I whispered "Get Dad" to my oldest daughter. Like a mountain climber, I moved one limb at a time as I slowly slid my body along the wall, the carpet pile scratching my cheek with each inching of my form. My children watched in horror as I slowly padded my way to the exit sign.

I vomited much of the night. When I could no longer crawl to the bathroom, I resorted to using the floor washing bucket. "Please help me, Lord," I cried over and over until I finally fell asleep sometime during the night.

Morning brought the sun. I opened my eyes and focused them on the light fixture above the bed. I slowly glanced to the door and then to the dresser and back to the light again. It seemed as though all was well. Perched on the side of the bed, I took a few moments to steady myself before standing up. I tried to piece together what had happened to me at the theater last night. I must have had a bout of food poisoning I concluded, but it might be best to call the doctor and make an appointment.

Over the course of the next few months, I went on to have many more of these attacks, averaging two to three a week. They were unpredictable. I would feel like myself one minute and the next minute I was looking for a place to lie down. Many times they would wake me in the early morning hours or begin with a headache in the evening, but at other times they were unannounced. After numerous medical tests, my diagnosis of Meniere's Disease left me confused and searching for answers.

I no longer felt independent or in control of my life. I was afraid to drive my children to their activities and would panic uncontrollably if I had to go somewhere alone, without my family. I sat at the end of the pew in church and I would mentally search out the exits and restrooms of every department store and restaurant. The bucket was now a permanent fixture under my bed. My purse was filled with peppermints, to ward off the bouts of nausea, and Valium to stop my head from spinning in circles once an attack had started. Life, as I knew it had been ripped out from under me and replaced with a life I did not understand, nor want. I did not know how to live in my new world.

I began to pray. I have always believed that God listens to us when we pray. We have only to reach out to Him. I have prayed for my family, my work, and for those who were hurting. But it was me who needed the prayers now. I needed God to stop these attacks, to comfort me until my world stopped spinning. So I prayed and prayed and prayed. I prayed in the morning when I woke up thanking God that I could get out of bed. I prayed in the evening to thank Him for getting me through another day without an attack of dizziness. I prayed when I felt the all too familiar queasiness begin and continued to pray throughout the long hours of the attacks. I whispered, shouted, and cried out in prayer.

God heard me.

As I recovered from each attack I began to see that I did have "good days". I stopped asking myself, why, and began to focus my attention on the lifestyle changes I needed to make. We purchased a low sodium cookbook and my husband and I learned to prepare meals with fresh herbs instead of salt. My family complained about the bland meals for a few weeks, but eventually learned to enjoy the taste of fresh vegetables and homemade breads. My husband and I made our nightly walks more of a priority, and I began to take a daily diuretic. I eventually asked for a different assignment at work and made sure that I received enough sleep each night in hopes of reducing stress. The changes I made are not only positive changes for me, but for my family as well.

I still suffer from attacks of Meniere's Disease and struggle with hearing loss, but over the last six years the attacks are not as frequent, nor as violent as before. I know the attacks can come at any time, but now I have the confidence to go ahead and make plans. I feel very blessed to have a doctor who understands this disease and helps me to live with my condition. I still stuff mints in my pockets and carry snacks in my purse for emergencies, but God helps me to cope and has given me the strength to go on with my life and not to be afraid. Even though there is no cure for this disease, through my faith and the support of my family He has given me the courage to fight it, but I am not fighting it alone.

Be still and know that I am God. –Psalm 46:10

THE WELCOME BASKET

Lisa McKhann

Once illness like cancer barges through the front door, the family inside never again steps back across that threshold quite the same. The street, the trees, the neighbors, the world stand forever askew. Though still familiar and recognizable, all perspective has collapsed. There is no unifying vantage point. Some things are so radically foreshortened as to lose all meaning. Others are over-burdened with Meaning. It's a world of icebergs and vertigo, megalomania and insomnia. Families shouldn't be left to squint, made nauseous by the brightness of daylight. Instead, they should find on the stoop this simple woven basket of goodies, something to carry to a dim, curtained space, to unpack and handle in privacy, your welcome basket.

On top, tucked under a silk or velvet ribbon, lies a printed greeting from the Neighborhood Welcome Committee with a list of neighbors' phone numbers. The fact that it's a form letter is to remind you that your family is not the only one living here in Cancerland or Crisistown. At first, this notion of having been joined up in some club of strangers may well offend you. Set aside your irritation and don't throw away the loathsome list. In your time, you may come to be grateful for others who navigate this alternate reality of illness. And farther down the road, you may put yourself on the call-list in someone else's basket.

There is a listing of three kinds of nearby services: the spiritual, the practical, and the official. For the spirit, area church services, of course, but also maybe tai chi and yoga, reiki and sand-play therapy. You will soon come to learn that meditation and silence are your friends, or so people say. Practical services begin with a local pharmacist, since anti-depressants and anxiety meds are an unspoken resource; then, neighbor kids who baby-sit, mow lawns, walk dogs (yes, pets feel the stress); an accountant to help you juggle your medical bills. You will wish it listed a personal injury lawyer to call; surely your illness is engaged in unlawful trespass. Finally, official services like the fire station, police, the ER. Your family will feel better knowing a few authority figures are on duty nearby. Everything is not lawless chaos. We have some civilizing elements. . . fire hydrants, for instance.

Your Welcome Basket includes a map of the emergency responders and of your own pressure relief valve: Nature. The map locates all the local parks where you can step onto dirt, not concrete; where you notice bird sounds, not traffic. Here you can see deep into layers of branches where the light is so subtle your eyes reach to distinguish color, your mind flits and rests lightly. On good days, you will trounce through your favorite park, invincible. On bad days, it will be a decent option, too.

Your basket undoubtedly contains a few offensively stupid things. Our sentiments are not always in sync. So, off to Goodwill with the plastic Jesus. And good will or good riddance to the false note like, "Wig shopping! Now you can be a blond!" Feel free to recycle these baubles and bobble-heads. What a relief to be able to act so decisively. Illness has arrived so for now, maybe forever, and certainly for better, you'll have less room for meaningless junk.

Done right, your basket includes an assortment of "Do Not Disturb" and "Keep Out" signs. For awhile, your family may find itself living in a gated community of sorts, where a guard holds a list of those who can pass, the rest politely yet firmly turned away. But without that, door-hangers are useful. "Do Not Disturbs" can be alternated with various forms of Welcome. "I'm In the Garden" sends visitors 'round back when you feel like fresh air and company. Your basket may include one cryptic sign, the FOYB sign. Not for public use, the foyb sign reminds you and your family to do only exactly what you want to do. For all else, no offense but, 'Fuck off, ya bastards'.

Ideally, your cancer basket will include one hand-made food item: cookies or, in the Midwest, maybe bars. An unsliced loaf of whole-wheat bread is ideal: hand-formed and miraculously risen, yet earthy, hearty and healthy—like you. This is the reminder that at core, your body is full of all the same sustaining powers.

If the Welcome Committee is on the ball, they will have included in your basket something for each member of your family. They will address even the cat or dog by name: a note about pick-up basketball with the guys; an invitation to stich-n-bitch with the girls; a request for kids to go sailing or join a bike ride; coupons to a local restaurant. Because, though whole families arrive here together, each individual moves through it in his or her unique way.

There will be a small, ribbon-tied bundle of thank-you cards in your basket. Because in this new neighborhood, you will find many opportunities to thank the people sharing their love in all kinds of ways. Someone will spend an afternoon on her knees weeding your perennial bed. And when you write her thank-you note, you will say what a relief, to see the peonies and tulips freed of entanglement. You will thank many people.

Way down at the very bottom, you will find a short, hand-written note. The message may say very little. Compared to the tangible specificity of the basket full of goodies and their associated uses, amid the very real stuff, words themselves stand in for meaning. They are space holders. A line or two in a person's own hand, *that* is the writing's power. Deep moments of contemplation lie behind the hand's most simply formed words, conjuring great love.

SOME WEIGHT

Kate Severson

"Why don't you just lose some weight?"

The words dug deep. She wasn't always this size. In her teens, she had been a scrawny anorexic, in her early twenties she weighed one hundred pounds. Those days she didn't watch what she ate because her daily Hershey bar supplemented her emotional and physical fuel.

The top button on her Levis pinched her stomach. She looked around for a rubber band to use as an extender.

"Why don't you just lose some weight?" Her husband asked a seemingly simple question one morning as they talked about her annoying sleep apnea. His question struck her soul. Her mental reply was that she was not overweight by choice. Her weight had evolved into a tense issue between them over the past couple of years, and it would take time to fix.

Not long ago, she walked several miles a week. She walked on her breaks, at lunch, on the weekend, savoring the feeling of her leg muscles tightening in transit and her breathing cycling through stages of respiration. Walking had been her moving meditation. The muscle toning made her feel fit not muscular like an athlete, but durable and strong. Her mobile addiction was as much for her spirit as for her muscles, but she could be fickle when the weather was too hot or too cold. She easily manufactured excuses to stay inside.

An accident suddenly sidelined her movement when a contractor's truck barreled into her car at full speed. The impact and concussion and muscle pain lingered for a long time. Her daily treks stopped and her legs were quick to soreness; because she wasn't used to walking, her muscles forgot how to behave.

She gained a few pounds—maybe even a couple of clothing sizes. She hoped that she could keep it a secret, but now and then her husband would comment about "their" need to go on a diet.

Suddenly, she faced another test when the breast cancer diagnosis changed her core. Weight and pain became incidental to cancer.

Surgery, radiation—these were her corporeal reality. Her weakened body could no more exercise than it could tell her whether the cancer remained in her cells.

But the next treatment phase proved to be the hardest. Hormones to fight the estrogen that her body had previously created and craved would turn against her. At first, the daily pills weren't tough to swallow because she was fighting cancer. Over the next several months, though, she was sore with every movement; her tender and swollen arms and legs and back kept her sitting through her lunch break instead of walking in the fresh air. Her mobility became a stationary mental stroll through words in books and scribbled text.

Her temperature came to a slow simmer three or four times an hour.

Sometimes, she rebelled against the pain and hot flashes and went for a walk, just like old times, but she paid for this energy spurt with a sore back and legs for the next week.

Her oncologist had predicted this. He offered an escalating chemical solution to her physical challenges—an endless loop through cancer therapy. She settled for a plan that would fight cancer but exacerbate her symptoms.

~~~~~~~

Her day begins with a costly cancer cocktail.

Is that her reflection? She notices her image in the mirror and wonders whether that is how people see her. Her profile belongs to a stranger; perhaps her weight gain is larger than she had realized. Her bumpy outline is prominent in every store window reflection she passes. Maybe, the next block will be more flattering. She walks with her breathe drawn, a balanced tepid tip-toe down the street.

She feels everyone's eyes on her stomach and her backside, their eyes denigrating her shape, her middle aged body disparaged by strangers.

What is that sour odor? Is that the scent of dogged fat cells or could it be cancer emitting its unrelenting presence?

She catches her husband's eye as they walk through the crowd. He looks too long at a woman walking by, justifying it by saying, "I like skinny!"

"Wow. Look at her!" He points out reedy women in the crowd and she feels like shrinking. His double takes remind her that her body is not his vision.

His ongoing irritation with her always comes back to some weight. Some weight that wasn't there a couple of years ago. Some weight that stands as the difference between svelte and squishy, some weight that serves as the wedge between harmony and heartburn.

The past two years have been too quick, too transformative, and too expansive.

A beautiful body showcased on "E!" keeps his eyes glued to the tube. His eyes sweep over the thin waist and tall slender legs and superficial plastic surgery on a trim body. He lingers over inane programs on other channels that showcase youth and skin.

She marks another evening with a liquid dinner. No unnecessary calories consumed tonight, except for that mood-relaxing glass of bitter beer.

Anna is his favorite server at the Salmon Head Brew Pub. Anna embodies his ideal, his slender and perfectly flawless vision. He stares at Anna as they sit at the bar, commenting on her skirt and shirt and boots and blonde hair that flips from side to side when she takes their order. Anna always has a benevolent sidewise smile for her, a silent ascent that she is aware of being watched, scrutinized; her pretty body on show for him and all of the other males in the room.

She could have exercised today. She didn't eat much, as usual, but work kept her too busy to walk into the snappy autumn Minnesota day. She'll indulge in hoppy beverages after work. She will tell him truthfully when he asks that she didn't eat dinner. He'll say "Good!" and remind her about losing some weight. He'll think that she is doing too little, too late, about her weight issue, but she feels the deprivation differently. The food isn't the point. Judgment doesn't nourish; it cultivates resentment with a lingering caustic aftertaste.

Her cancer has provided her with new opportunities for confronting her emotional landscape. She takes in the unforeseen dips and peaks with a relative acceptance that comes with age, a tolerance that she couldn't have summoned in her anorexic youth. Her current body is only a detached likeness; her spirit is in transition.

She has been offered several cancer resource lists, but her most courageous task is to ask for help and accept emotional aid. She vows to make some cautious inquiries into the vast survivorship network. Her friends ask how she is doing. She will try to tell them her true feelings about cancer treatment. Authenticity will be her therapeutic and spiritual healing.

Tomorrow she'll walk. If not tomorrow, then sometime next week. She'll walk at lunch, and will hope that this is the start of a new routine. She'll feel the toning in her calves and will pledge to walk again the next day. She'll reflect on her healing and her trials as she walks in defiance of some weight.

JESKE NOORDERGRAAF

My love of animals is a part of me. Thinking back to the Christmas' of my childhood, all I ever wanted was a pony. I did not dream about a storybook wedding but instead about riding a horse over the high and colorful jumps during the Olympics. I wasn't a good enough equestrian to make this dream come true especially with my parents requiring that I go to college so I chose a different path but one that still kept me with horses. I became a veterinarian.

There have been obstacles during my life but the Olympic sized one came into my life on December 5, 2005, when my routine mammogram was abnormal. A mass was found in one of my breasts and my life changed. I started the day feeling great and ended the day concerned that I was going to die. Instead of being the one treating the illness, I was the patient and my life was in other hands.

The most difficult part of the original diagnosis was the waiting. Yes, there was an abnormality but was it cancerous and if it was cancerous had it spread and what type was it. Just like learning to walk, each step was slow and the waiting for results was tough especially when it led to yet another test. Christmas is a time to rejoice but in 2005 it was challenging as I didn't want to upset my family while I endured test after test. I could not just say, oh it is nothing when chances were that it was significant.

In the New Year, I finally was ready to start treatment after the type of cancer had been determined. Although the last month had been emotionally draining, physically I still felt great. Now I was going to get sick so I could get better. And how was I going to manage my family and business. I was married and had an eight-year-old son. I also owned my own veterinary practice, had employees and felt responsible for them. So being the goal oriented person I am, I made a list of my priorities and started my treatment.

I wanted my son's life to be as normal as possible; I did not want this to be what defined his childhood. Of course, I was going to do what my doctors recommended but I was going to try to keep my life as positive as I could. Although one doctor had told me early on that I would need to take six months off from my practice, I did not want to do this. My dream after giving up on the Olympics was to be a veterinarian and specialize in the care of horses and that is what I was doing. At the time that all this was happening, one associate had unexpectedly left to pursue his dream and I was already shorthanded. I could not just abandon my clients and give up. Also, I felt that work was a good distraction as I was unable to dwell on my problems while working on a twelve-hundred pound horse who might not feel that I needed to treat him.

I did keep working and arranged my chemotherapy around weekends. I wore a wig for a few weeks but it was always slipping so I decided a hat was a better option for me. I had a supportive and compassionate medical team on my side. My family and friends were essential both for the logistics of getting to medical appointments and for showing they care. I know how hard it is to ask someone who is ill or having a challenging time how they are doing. Does the person asking just want to hear fine, or does he or she really care. Even though it can't change the outcome, every positive word of encouragement and demonstration of concern feels like a pat on the back and I do believe that a positive attitude can help. I kept every card I received and hung them up to act as encouragement.

At the beginning of my treatment, I was not sure that I was going to survive. My husband, son and I had been attending a local church but were not members. I decided to join at this time as the church community was very supportive and I wanted to be a true part of the church. I like to tell people that I joined when I did because it would save money on the cost of the funeral. This always made people laugh, making a serious problem more manageable.

There were other positives along the way. I finally learned how to use makeup when I went to the American Cancer Society's look good feel better class. Also, my hair grew back curly and blond with highlights and my mother told me that I was prettier than before. I saved money on haircuts and shampoos and my skin was the clearest it had ever been.

I was fortunate enough to survive my cancer but the disease is never gone. It remains with me as a reminder that it could come back. Both when I take my daily medication and when I get dressed—the reminders are there. I visit my oncologist semi-annually which is a confidence booster. Has the disease changed me besides physically? It has, I am more understanding and compassionate. No one really knows what is going on in someone else's life. I am thankful that I survived, that my family is intact and that my son is growing up to be compassionate. Also, I am appreciative of all my clients who asked how I was doing and understood that some days were hard and that I had to limit what I could do.

JUST BEYOND THE DOOR

Dorothy Sauber

It's been decades since my body felt the press of imminent danger. One cold, moonless January night in a Minnesota town on the Canadian border, I entered the front door of a friend's empty dark house and heard what I thought was a hungry wolf howling in the alley out back. As I hung up my wool coat, the howling and wailing grew louder and moved closer. Once I'd followed the sounds to the rear of the house, I discovered the desperate creature had begun clawing its way through the door.

It had broken through the door's outer wooden layer and was in a frenzy to finish the job. By the time help arrived, I was exhausted from holding my body as counterweight against the thrusting force on the other side. My friend's father appeared just in time to help save the door from the ramming lunges of the raging animal. More help arrived in the form of the local cop. While the two of us inside were using our combined strength to keep the animal from snapping the metal lock open, a shot rang out. One well-aimed bullet from the cop's gun quieted the roaring mass of muscle outside the door. With his flashlight on high beam, the cop showed us the foaming mouth and crazed eyes of a very large, very dead, rabid dog.

Years later, on another cold, dark January night in Minnesota, I find myself holding my full weight against another door. But unlike that scary night long ago, I know all too well that this time around the bullet aimed to kill the crazed creature has major limitations. And what separates me from certain danger is even thinner than a hollow oak door.

Thirteen months ago today I was diagnosed with Stage IV lung cancer. The average life expectancy for this kind of cancer is one year. That I have reached this average life expectancy still in good health and high spirits is due in large part to a newly approved wonder drug I've been taking faithfully at four P.M. every day since my first visit with the oncologist.

At the end of every visit, however, my oncologist never fails to look me in the eye and say, "One day this drug you are taking will stop working." I hear his words. I take in their significance and resolve to hold even firmer to every day of life for the gift it is. Then I go back to my life as I have been living it this past year. I return to my full schedule of lunches with friends, I go to the movies, I plan trips to visit my sons, and I think of myself as being mighty lucky to be mingling still among the living.

But tonight I learned that the rabid dog of cancer may have moved closer to my door. I just finished reading, *Lung Cancer: Not Just for Smokers*, in the *Harvard Health Letter*. The article includes information about the new "smart" drug I take every day and which I have been counting on to keep me, not just healthy, but alive. "Virtually all patients who respond to these drugs develop resistance within fourteen months or so." Patient resistance to this pioneer cancer therapy drug has put the damper on their promise. That I am only one month away from another grave marker in the lung cancer study statistics makes me hear again what sounds like the howls of a hungry wolf just beyond the door.

Every morning I scan the obituaries feeling grateful I am still reading the obituaries. If there is one thing I have learned this past year, it is that until any of us is actually dead, life within our hearts and minds is relentless in pushing on. For the first time, I see my own pulsing greed for living. I want more life: I want one more month, one more year, one more day to be here where I so love being. I want to keep breathing and smelling and tasting until there is no air or lavender or honey left anywhere on the planet.

Ruth Picardie, a British journalist and the mother of one-year-old twins, was diagnosed with breast cancer when she was thirty-two-years-old and died a month after her twins' second birthday. She left behind a wonderfully frank record of how she dealt with her cancer, how others treated her, and what she saw as the injustices of her own death. She wrote in *Before I Say Goodbye,* "After a fourth acquaintance tells you their aunt has breast cancer, you realize you don't feel sorry for any postmenopausal woman who has the disease because fifty-something isn't a bad crack at life, especially if your kids have grown up."

Ruth died too young to know that, with very few exceptions, most people, regardless of their age or physical condition, long for death to extend its deadline by a few weeks or years or decades. There might be a wedding coming up or a family reunion. Grandchildren are born, and we want to hear them talk and watch them go off to college.

Being greedy about life is a most basic human condition. But I never knew just how greedy I was until the door separating me from death cracked open. As often as I tell myself I have had a better chance than many by living this long and this well, I still don't want to die. Like a snake-oil saleswoman talking out of both sides of her mouth, I remind myself that we all must die, and I can die today satisfied I have had a good life. Then my other voice chimes in to tell me I have all the time in the world yet to laugh, love, and linger over afternoon tea with a friend.

Ruth Picardie was right to feel she was missing out on a lot of life by dying young. I know I would not want to have missed seeing my own children grow up and have children of their own. I'm glad I survived long enough to have my loved ones here several weeks ago singing Christmas carols. And I'm grateful I lived to go to the bookstore yesterday to add to my winter reading pile.

I certainly had no say about getting lung cancer. Now I have no say about how long this wonder drug will work. But I can continue to fill my lunch plate with raw beets, carrots, and broccoli, stay off white sugar, drink plenty of water, swallow my four P.M. pill and boil up my Chinese acupuncturist's herbal medicines. The last time she studied my tongue and measured the life force in both my wrists, the acupuncturist said, "You have less heat. Better inside than before." It turns out that less heat inside is good for whatever ails us. And in spite of menacing sounds just beyond the door, less heat might just be all I need to get to savor a little more of life.

KRIS BRENNA LYONS

"Don't worry about it. It's probably nothing."

Take a test. Test comes back.

"Don't worry about it. It's probably nothing."

That is what the medical personnel keep saying. Take another test. Test comes back.

"Don't worry about it. It's probably nothing."

Take still another test. Test comes back.

Well, they are wrong, all wrong.

It IS something!

We have had no breast cancer on my mother's side. I wasn't really worried. Then words in the doctor's office are thrown about, such as, "fine needle biopsy," "get clean margins," "ductal carcinoma in situ," "estrogen receptor positive," and more mention by doctors of types of "opsies" and "ectomies" until the overload on the brain is about to erupt.

I know many women journal every moment what happened and how they felt with this life changing news. I didn't have a clue as to any concrete thoughts, just rolling emotions or disbelief. I was stunned and mortified and frightened. My best friend and I use to joke about whom was losing body parts faster: a gall bladder here, some knee cartilage there, crack a tooth, crown a tooth…whatever.

We'd have a little contest and goad one another about losses. This was different. This would be an actual body part I see and then: cut, sliced, diced, and gone! It wasn't so humorous anymore. I really didn't want to lose this particular contest, not this way.

How could this happen? I guess it had to do with the following: I had had a complete hysterectomy a year earlier and was prescribed estrogen. Lots of women do that. I, also, remember when I was hit in the chest as an umpire by a pitch in girls fast pitch softball when the catcher didn't even attempt to put her glove up to catch the ball. Of course, I was not wearing a chest protector. I was blue and deep purple and later green and yellow in the whole breast area and beyond. Blunt trauma force probably not good for the bod either. Sometimes, women who have been in car accidents and have hit the dashboards with their chests later have breast cancer diagnoses, too. I would guess this trauma is similar. The point is *life happens.*

A cyst was originally spotted on my yearly mammogram. We were going to take a biopsy to be sure what it was. The medical woman accidentally ran the guide wire into the cyst. The cyst was gone! I had to wait another six months to see if it would return. This was the first time those reassuring words were stated, "Don't worry about it. It's probably nothing." The cyst did return. So whether the sun, the moon, and the stars all lined up with positive receptors, blunt force trauma, genetics, no genetics, I got the bad news. It was cancer!

We did it all: a biopsy, a lumpectomy, and a mastectomy. I was diagnosed with ductal carcinoma situ that was sprayed out like a shotgun into the breast. I sobbed. It's funny how one gets attached to body parts even if one just takes them for granted. Options were given. Decisions had to be made.

It was summer and I was golfing in a local league with Marilyn who was in her late 70s. She said she had heard my upsetting news. As the two of us walked together across the course in a very open area with a view from the clubhouse, she all of a sudden stopped and released the handle of her golf cart. She abruptly grabbed her right breast and shook it a little bit. Then she grabbed her left breast and did the same. Next she pulled her blouse a way from her body and peaked down the front of the blouse at her breasts.

"Aw, hell. I can't remember any more which one I lost unless I really think about it." I started to giggle and then belly laugh at her incredible actions on the golf course. She did the same. Marilyn shared with me *her* story. She told how difficult it was in the late 60s with chemo and radiation. She had young sons at the time, too. She said medical techniques and treatment are way better today. I would be just fine.

From that point on, I knew I would be successful in beating this beast because of Marilyn's uninhibited actions on a golf course one day. It was her unselfishness in sharing a cancer story that got me through to the acceptance of my own cancer, treating it, and moving on to face whatever the future would hold. I had come to terms with this dark companion. I would face it as others have before me and will after me until it's cured.

Incidentally, I just celebrated my fifth cancer free anniversary. Thanks, Marilyn.

CAROL A SCHREIER

The subtle pressure in my abdomen woke me. "If it's not gone in a week I'll go in," I told myself. It wasn't and I did. A good friend of mine had ovarian cancer, so I was well informed. I knew what to ask for: a vaginal ultra-sound. I also had two physicians who responded immediately to my concerns. Five days later I was in surgery. The outcome: ovarian cancer, clear cell type. FIGO, Stage 1-A.

"If I die from this, do not put 'I lost my valiant battle with cancer' in my obituary," I told my daughter. The war metaphor offended me. The cancer was mine; this process of out-of-control, crazy-growth-gone-wild was part of me. I worked hard to accept this. I engaged my mind and body, every physical and spiritual resolve of my being to befriend this cancer; all the while wanting it not to be.

I determined to do everything my western medical doctors suggested and to research and do everything a more holistic approach deemed helpful. I had surgery and chemotherapy. I drank an awful, noxious concoction of tea made of twigs, seed and leaves prescribed by an herbalist. I boiled the ingredients three times before drinking. I changed my diet and included shitaki mushrooms, blueberries and a variety of food containing anti-oxidants. I had weekly massages. I did QI Gong daily.

I meditated daily on the inevitability of aging, illness, and death. I used a meditation suggested to me by a Buddhist friend. It began, "I am of the nature to grow old. There is no way to escape growing old. I am of the nature to have ill health. There is no way to escape having ill health. I am of the nature to die. There is no way to escape death. All that is dear to me and everyone I love are of the nature to change. There is no escape being separated from them. My deeds are my closest companions I am the beneficiary of my deeds. My deeds are the ground on which I stand." This meditation gradually informed my life and my activities.

I consulted a former therapist. I talked of my terror at not existing, of not having conscious awareness of my existence. He reminded me that every night when I went to sleep I gave up conscious awareness.

"Will I ever not think of my cancer all the time?" I asked a friend. She was a two-time survivor of breast cancer, a clear-headed, direct-spoken, Dutch woman. "If you survive, and 'if' is the operative word, you will find yourself on a train for which you did not buy a ticket and from which you cannot disembark. When you arrive at your destination, you will find yourself in an exotic locale where you do not speak the language and do not understand the customs. That is the journey, and your task is to find your place again. And, yes, if you do survive the cancer, the anxiety will subside."

I relied on the kindness of family and friends, I lived alone, but for the first three months following my diagnosis I did not cook a meal. Friends brought lovingly prepared food with enough for additional meals; they stocked my larder. They prayed for me.

A niece who taught second grade in a Catholic elementary school where daily prayers and specific intentions were part of the routine added my name. Her students asked who I was and she told them I was her aunt, about to have surgery. They prayed for me and wrote me letters, "do not worry, I've had surgery, too", and, "do not be afraid."

Part of my healing journey included facilitating an ovarian cancer support group. A group member asked, "how do you deal with the anxiety that comes unbidden at 4:00 A.M.?" Everyone shared. One woman said she treated it the same way she treated a new rattle in her car, "I turn the radio up."

"And you," they asked me, "what do you do?" I said I imagined a wide circle of people in pain that spread like ripples in a pond.

I prayed first for my closest neighbors and then expanded to the block and the neighborhood. I included specific people who were hurting in the larger community. As I prayed, I calmed. The sweat dried on my skin. My heart slowed and reclaimed its rightful place inside my skin.

I went to church and wept during the music played following communion. As an adult I had stopped attending the Catholic Church. A friend invited me to visit her church. There was something about this church and this priest who preached only the love of God that was healing. I determined to attend until the weeping ceased. I went weekly for one year.

As my friend had predicted, my cancer anxiety subsided but slowly, very slowly. For the first three years, I had a CA-125 test measuring a protein present in the blood every three months. This test, while not a reliable indicator for an initial diagnosis, is reliable in tracking reoccurrences. After three years, I went on a once-every-six-months schedule for two years. Currently, I am seen once a year. There has been no evidence of a reoccurrence. I am lucky. I had the benefit of my friends' experience, excellent physicians, and adequate health insurance.

Did this experience, this journey, change me? Of course it did. How could it not? It was a struggle but not against an alien intruder. The struggle was an internal one, the only kind that really matters, a struggle to accept and befriend my own body, my own illness, my own human frailty; to harness whatever healing was possible, to accept death if my healing journey included death. It hasn't for the past thirteen years but it will...someday.

Coming To Terms

When cancer comes, the universe shifts; the mind snaps to attention.
The soul struggles for balance, grieving, giving, reaching out, receiving,
placing one foot before the other with purposeful intention,
to accept, to breathe, to live.

Original poem by Carol A. Schreier

MARY ALICE HARROLD

I have come to terms with the dark companion of my illness of Bipolar II, Mixed, Most Recent Episode Depressed, with Psychotic Features. I was diagnosed when I was twenty-six years old and a first year law student. The onset of this Serious and Persistent Mental Illness (SPMI) can be triggered while an individual is under inordinate amounts of stress. That was the case with me that dark and ugly winter of 1989.

The frenzied mania came in the fall of that year. I was unable to sleep, had difficulty concentrating, couldn't complete tasks, and was spending inordinate amounts of money. I was irritable with others, irrationally angry, and talked fast and constantly. The psychosis began when I started having delusions that the "FBI" was trailing me because my mother hired the "agents" to place me on a mental health unit. I also was delusional and paranoid about the thoughts of others. I felt terrified all of the time.

I went into the lobby of the Hyatt Hotel in Minneapolis and spent the remainder of the day and evening sitting in a chair too terrified to go outside. The "FBI" might apprehend me and whisk me away to a regional treatment center for years to come.

The day at the Hyatt was the most dark, terrifying, and lonely day of my life. I was asked by the doorman to leave the hotel and an ambulance was waiting outside to take me to the Hennepin County Medical Center in Minneapolis.

I was placed on a locked unit with patients who had lost touch with reality as I had. I was transferred to United Hospital in St. Paul as the county facility did not have an available bed for me. I was restrained in the van by an orderly and felt like a prisoner who had committed a crime.

I was admitted to the hospital and it was a long and arduous process. I was roomed at two in the morning and given medication I thought was part of the "FBI" plot to imprison me. A psychiatrist reassured me that the medication would take away the fear I was feeling. I did not believe her, but, did comply with taking the medications.

The next morning, I met with a psychiatrist who had arranged for my mother to come to the unit to meet with us to discuss my case. My mother accused me of doing horrible things during my mania. She told me I was a "psychiatric mess" and needed to be committed to a state hospital. I became afraid and angry with her that led me to begin screaming and crying uncontrollably. The psychiatrist and the hospital put me on a commitment order as a result. This meant I was under the control of the legal system until I complied with my treatment plan and began recovering from my mania.

If I took my medication, met with the psychiatrist, and attended all hospital groups I would be placed on a stay of commitment. I would then meet with a judge who would decide if any treatment upon discharge was appropriate.

I spent two weeks in the hospital and was placed on Lithium as a mood stabilizer and Zyprexa for the psychotic symptoms. Within two weeks, I was feeling stronger and more mentally stable.

I went to court and the judge placed me on a stay of commitment. I was ordered to attend an out-patient program five days a week to continue working towards recovery. I agreed to take my medication and work with a new psychiatrist and therapist as well.

Upon discharge from the hospital, I felt the darkness of depression wash over me like the pouring rain. I had no energy, poor concentration, feelings of hopelessness, low self esteem, and suicidal thoughts.

My psychiatrist added an anti-depressant to my medication plan and I took it religiously. I was tortured by loneliness, negative thoughts/feelings, and the inability to focus on my treatment goals. My family was concerned seeing the variations of my moods. I was in an intense manic state and then suddenly became depressed.

My depression has not responded to a succession of anti-depressants taken over the last twenty-five years. I still feel its strength and power every day of my life. I isolate myself and feel a deep sadness most of the time. It is a monster in my life. My dark companion never leaves me. I can only try to manage it on a daily basis.

On the other hand, my manic episodes have been treated successfully and I have never had a manic episode since 1989. I have never had to live with that terror again and for that I am grateful.

I have suffered from having this disorder. Being on mood stabilizers has caused me to gain over one hundred and fifty pounds since 1989. I am ashamed of this and disappointed in the way I look physically now. I don't want others to see that I have grown from a fit and active person into three hundred pounds of obesity.

I also have lost many friends due to isolating myself. I don't return their phone calls, e-mails, texts, or letters.

I was unable to work for twelve years and received Social Security Disability payments. I was deemed as being disabled by my Bipolar Disorder and needed to receive benefits. My family has also suffered from the "run-off" of my disorder. I couldn't take care of myself and my apartment when I was disabled and unemployed.

There are blessings and curses of having Bipolar Disorder. I am intelligent and did well in school. I attended one year of law school and was successful in my classes despite having a manic episode during my first semester.

This was also the year that my father developed cancer. He was treated, moved to a hospice, and passed away. I did not return to law school the next year because I started to decompensate after his death and was awarded Social Security benefits once again.

I have positive relationships with my mother and siblings now. I am grateful for the love, support, and guidance I receive from my family.

I am active in the Native communities in Minneapolis and White Earth Minnesota. I am a member of the White Earth Band of Ojibwe. I have met fellow writers and artists during the last two years and have a greater knowledge of my culture. I am also starting classes during the summer to learn my native Ojibwe language.

I belong to a native writer's group, a native women's book club, and a weekly writing group. I see a trainer and am trying to lose weight and become fit again. I have lost thirty pounds since the first of this year.

My mother had open heart surgery and I did not fall apart as I would have in the past. I am in control of my feelings, thoughts, and reactions to life events.

I have an excellent medical team including a psychiatrist, therapist, weekly group, and all of the socializing that sustains me. I know I can count on my friends and they can rely on me. I am less isolated now and my depressed mood has improved greatly.

I have held the same job as a social service Case Manager for six years. I recently had a good job review with my supervisor and received another raise in income this year. I have accepted my dark companion and the trials and tribulations it has brought into my life. I have learned a lot from this writing experience but have relived some uncomfortable feelings and memories. Thank you for the opportunity to be part of this wonderful writing project to honor the memory and strength of Kelly Culhane.

CAROL LARSON

I don't have to go back very far to recall when I learned to live again.

Twelve years ago, I knew something was wrong. My husband and I were driving to a party just two weeks before Christmas. I was looking out the window onto a scene of powdered meringue snowdrifts, thinking, *Minnesota is a beautiful place to live*. At that moment, I had an eerie revelation: if I wanted to see another winter, I needed to check out some suspicious signs I had been ignoring. I turned to my husband, Dave.

"Could we stop at Urgent Care before we go to the party?"

"Now?" he said, perplexed. I rarely went to a doctor. "Are you sick?"

"I'm not sure, but I might be." I explained how tired I had been feeling and that I had experienced minor spotting, thinking it might be hemorrhoids. Only, I was pretty certain that wasn't the trouble. It might be something worse.

When the doctor at Urgent Care finally examined me, my worst fears were confirmed. This was not going to be an easy fix.

"Any kind of unexplained bleeding is a red flag. You need to call a doctor on Monday morning and schedule a colonoscopy. Don't let them lose any time getting you in."

Within a few days, I had completed the irksome prep, ready for my exam.

Two polyps were discovered and removed painlessly. The doctor said they looked benign, but he needed to test them with a biopsy. He promised to call me when he got the test results back, and I was sent home with optimism.

In fact, I was so relieved, that I didn't even consider in the following week how much I was tying up our phones using our dial-up computer. On December twenty-fourth, I got a call from the gastroenterologist who had done the colonoscopy.

"Mrs. Larson, I'm sorry to call you on this day, but I've been trying to get hold of you for the last two days and I really need to give you this news." His voice was apologetic, but insistent. "One of the polyps we biopsied turned out to be malignant. I'm hoping we got it all in surgery during the colonoscopy, but I want to refer you to a colorectal surgeon immediately." I was stunned. I didn't want to believe what I was hearing.

Nevertheless, I did call, and had the good fortune to get an excellent colorectal surgeon. One of the best. After examining me, he confirmed the diagnosis of rectal cancer Stage One. Just to make sure, he sent me to one of his partners for periodic ultra-sounds. Two months later, when that doctor was examining me with an endoscope, we watched the results on a screen. The room became very quiet. The only sound was the beeping of the machine announcing bad news. The doctor's silence told me he was reluctant to tell me what he was seeing: Three dark invaders showed up where they shouldn't be. When he started to plot quadrants over them, I succumbed to despair. My body stiffened. In a sympathetic, soft voice, he said, "I'm sorry. It looks like the cancer has spread to your lymph nodes."

My heart was racing from adrenaline running through my veins.

"I have to cut off a little of each node to have it biopsied," he apologized.

His snipping didn't hurt, really. I wasn't feeling any physical pain but was filled with dread as we discussed my future.

"If the tests come out positive, you're going to need a resection, radiation, and chemotherapy."

I held back tears; I tried to respond, to organize my thoughts, my life by groping for the familiar, the old routines I desperately wanted to protect me. "But I can't do that at this point." It was a shaky plea for more time. "My daughter, Laura is getting married this summer."

He wasn't buying any of it. Solemnly he said, "You need to take care of your health first, you know."

What he was saying made sense. My life had taken a momentous turn. To deny the danger would be the worst course of action I could take.

Still, I found myself fighting facts. I spent the next two days in suspended belief waiting for the final results to come in. I suspected I was in deep trouble, but I wasn't going to accept that fact until I actually knew for sure. Waiting in itself is a challenge for one's ability to withstand anxiety. It is, in some ways, worse than the actual ordeal. More than anything else, I wanted the waiting to be over.

At 9:00 AM the phone rang. It was from my doctor who had done the ultrasound. Cancer had spread to my lymph nodes. He would call my colorectal surgeon immediately. I weakly replied I understood what he was saying. He ended the conversation by telling me with conviction, "I want you to know we're going to fight this." I hung up the phone and faced the truth. The good health I had taken for granted had broken down. My life was rerouted on a momentous detour. I had to get major repairs in order to survive.

At a moment like this, you need a champion. In the past, my brother took on this role for me. I called him and he came over immediately. I was sobbing and he let me do that. He reminded me that in our genetic pool, many of our relatives had cancer and survived. Rationality entered the picture and I started to settle down. I had cancer that had metastasized into my lymph nodes. So what? I was going to have to endure some aggressive measures if I was going to live. I wasn't denying this fact anymore. This was to be my dark companion for the next year, but I lost some of my fear. My way of handling any crisis took over. I came to terms with it, and that grounded me. From then on, I was determined to learn all I could how to cope with cancer.

I have just finished my twelfth Christmas since then. It hasn't all been easy and there have been some setbacks. At those times, I've prayed for strength. My faith, family, and friends have contributed to my recovery. Support groups and staying away from negative stress have empowered me. Through the years, memories of my detour with cancer have faded. Some of that is good because life goes on.

I never want to forget some of the lessons I've learned because they have made me a more experienced traveler, leaving illness behind and looking ahead to new destinations. Although this was not the trip I had planned to take, I have a new outlook on life: to be more appreciative of the ordinary aspects of life that I used to take for granted.

BRENDA MARTIN-GRANSTRA

I always thought of myself as strong and healthy. I didn't get sick often and seldom missed work. I was the type to go to work regardless of how I was feeling because I felt my job needed to get done and it was easier than making someone else come in—and because I felt guilty about using a sick day and getting paid for staying home. I also thought I was lucky or blessed or otherwise immune from what strikes so many others. Would you call that optimistic? Or superior? So even before the diagnosis, with all the extra appointments, I felt guilty that I would be missing work with extra appointments and embarrassed that I was one of "those" people who got sick and would be making my employer pay for sick days.

There was a long list of things I considered that might have caused my illness. Was it environmental carcinogens, or excess weight? Could birth control pills have brought it on, or was it an inactive lifestyle? Was it stress or refilling plastic water bottles? Friday night happy hours and the "social" smoking that used to go with it? Microwave popcorn? My addiction to sunflower seeds? I wondered if God had abandoned me. But how could I have it both ways, when I had been struggling with my faith anyway in the years leading up to this?

A nurse navigator told me that I was on a "journey." Now I can see that a navigator can be a comfort to a newly diagnosed, scared cancer patient, but when I was yet in disbelief, I found it annoying—just give me the facts and stay away from my feelings. Don't make me cry. And this "journey?"—I'd rather just take a trip.

Dozens of times every day, when the situation came to mind again, after the disbelief, my stomach would drop and I would feel heartsick. And it wasn't so much that I was thinking I was going to die—it was just the thought that I had a disease. That I had been judged or would be judged. Then, returning from another appointment, a thought occurred to me: *People get cancer. People just get cancer. They just do.*

When that idea hit me, a feeling came over me that seemed like the saying of "peace that passes understanding." It was like being struck with a grace stick that gave instant relief. I wasn't convinced that I was going to be okay. I didn't know without a doubt that everything would turn out all right, but at least the burden of self incrimination was lifted. I went from denial to acceptance in a quarter of a mile.

Ever since I was about thirty, I had related to the John Mellencamp song with the verse that goes: "Life goes on long after the thrill of living is gone." Already ten or fifteen years ago, I would find myself thinking, "I'm still here. I'm still alive. So much time has passed, so many have passed before me. So much has changed and yet life goes on. I wonder how long?" What will be, will be. Is that being a fatalist?

I don't think I'll be afraid to die if that's the way this goes, but I don't want to not live well or not die well, if that is possible. I didn't think I'd get cancer the first time—now I guess anything is possible. I don't think I'd be surprised. But the sinking feeling, if there is a next time; I believe will have more to do with the mortality and fear of diminishing returns than in what others may think.

I thought, "It could be worse...." I've lived the best part of my life. My kids are grown—they will be okay. So I've been telling people to do what it is they really want to do, because you never know when life is going to hand you a smack down.

I'm kind of a loner. I like to think I can do things on my own. I was surprised, a little embarrassed, and humbled by the number of people in my community who called, sent cards and gifts, and offered to cook, clean, and drive for me and my family.

Some women are just long-hair types. I hadn't had short hair since I was in grade school. I always thought my ears and nose were too big, so I used long hair to hide in. About a month before chemo started, I had my hair cut short and it wasn't as bad as I thought.

Next, I was afraid of how ugly my bald head would look—I'd always felt I had a long, narrow face and a ridge on top of my head. I called where my hair parted, oh, so naturally, the Great Divide. When I was showering soon after chemo started, I found myself pushing fallen hair away from the drain with my foot. That same day I had my husband buzz my head. Again, not as bad as I feared.

After a while, I complained to my husband that the mangy stubble left on my head made me look worse than sick. I said, "It makes me look..." and my dear husband filled in, "Like you have a disease?" I feigned indignation and we both laughed. And then I used an extra sticky lint roller and got the rest of the patches of stubble off my head.

There were a few issues with treatments, but I made it through with everyone's help. Now, I am waiting for the follow-up with the oncologist—I guess I could consider it the waiting game, but I hope to not dwell too much on what may come. I know it helps to have something; anything to do that brings you satisfaction and takes your mind off the dark cloud over your shoulder. It has also been helpful to try not to worry about what others may think of your appearance and to laugh at some of the absurdities. For instance, I knew it was time to give up the wig when it had gotten cold and I found myself tugging down on both sides like it was a stocking cap.

LIKE MOTHER, LIKE DAUGHTER

Joy Riggs

My fourteen-year-old daughter breezes through the door, dumps her overnight bag on the floor and finds me in the kitchen.

"It's just not fair, Mom," Louisa says. "Why do girls have to go through this?"

I guess—correctly—that she got her period during the night and had not packed supplies.

She looks at me with mischief in her hazel eyes. "To make it fair, I think boys should be kicked in the nuts once a month."

I smile at this proposal, and I make a mental note to warn her twelve-year-old brother, Sebastian, that this might not be the day to attempt to engage her in one of his monologues about the prowess of Greek and Roman soldiers. At least, not without a protective shield.

Louisa explains that she wasn't able to sleep because of cramps.

"It felt like there was a balloon expanding in my stomach, and I couldn't get comfortable," she says.

For a second, my thoughts flash back to my own early years of menstruation, when I'd feel a twisting pain in my abdomen and wonder, *is this what it feels like to have a baby*?

I realize Louisa is looking at me expectantly, waiting for reassurance. I consider telling her the truth. My truth. If things go as I expect, my days of menstruating will soon cease. I will have my ovaries surgically removed to prevent them from killing me. I also am contemplating a preventive mastectomy.

But I'm not ready to talk about all that, so I shift into sensible mom mode.

"I had cramps at your age, too, but I don't get them anymore. It will get better," I say. "If the cramps are still bothering you, you could take some Motrin."

Satisfied with this response, she goes upstairs to her bedroom, and my thoughts return to the phone call I received a few days earlier.

The counselor's warm but professional voice informed me that I'd inherited my mom's genetic mutation. It meant I had a much higher likelihood of developing breast and ovarian cancer over my lifetime than women without the mutation. Specifically, women with a BRCA1 mutation have a sixty to eighty percent lifetime risk for breast cancer, compared to the general population risk of twelve percent. For ovarian cancer, they have a twenty to forty percent risk, compared to the general risk of one to two percent.

My stomach dropped. It was the answer I'd come to expect, but it was not what I wanted to hear.

"The risk was there before you took the test; now, you can do something about it," the counselor said.

I tried to respond with lines I'd rehearsed in my head in case of this result. My airway felt clogged.

"It's good to finally know," I managed to say, my voice quavering.

The counselor said that I should take time to let it sink in, and that it was okay to feel sad. She reminded me that options existed to reduce my risks.

"You're in the generation creating the change in mindset. It will be easier for your kids, and for your nieces and nephews," she said.

Ah, yes. That was one reason I'd finally decided to take the test. Did my kids have the mutation, too? Louisa was the only one with ovaries, but the boys could be carriers and face greater risk for male breast cancer and prostate cancer.

The counselor reviewed my next steps—getting an MRI scan of my breasts, and meeting with a doctor to discuss oophorectomy, a surgery to remove my ovaries. I'd already decided I wanted the surgery if I had the mutation because it could reduce my risk of ovarian cancer by eighty to ninety-six percent.

"You can pick a time that works with your family schedule," she said. "Being young and healthy, you're going to recover quickly."

I silently thanked her for the young comment; the news had me feeling older than forty-three. I wanted to tell my mom immediately, but I knew I wouldn't be able to get the words out. So I sent her an email.

Fifteen years earlier, when I was newly pregnant with Louisa, we'd found out that Mom had something growing inside her, too—a mass of cancerous cells. Stage III ovarian cancer. One of her sisters had died from the disease, and the other sister had battled breast cancer. What my mom taught me through her long recovery—and what she still shows me, as an active woman in her seventies—is that love can carry you through pain and fear to a place of unexpected blessings. Where would my journey take me?

Mom's concise email response indicated that she was taking the news hard—she, the woman who would bring me cold washcloths when I was younger and say, "I wish I could be sick instead of you," as though by saying it she could transfer the fever from my body to hers. I knew that, as much as she wanted to, she could not fix this.

I didn't feel composed enough to call her until late that evening, once the kids were in bed. She answered on the first ring.

"Hi, Mom," I said brightly.

I wanted to set the right tone, and let her know I was okay.

"I was so sorry to get your news. I just didn't think you had it," she said. She sounded tired and sad.

"Well, I thought I had it. I guess I've thought that for a long time. It does feel good to finally know, after all this time of wondering, because now I can do something about it."

My voice sounded optimistic, unwaveringly positive. I hoped I sounded the same to her. Mom did well—she only choked up once, when she mentioned telling a close friend the news, and she had to hand the phone to my dad for a few minutes.

When I got off the phone, I felt lighter. Having a mutation sounded scary, but it didn't mean getting cancer was inevitable. I could take preventive actions to benefit myself and my kids.

I slept soundly that night.

My feelings of empowerment increased the next day when I discussed the news with my friend Carrie.

"Okay, you inherited your mom's genetic mutation, but she's a survivor, right? I bet you also inherited her survivor gene," Carrie said confidently.

I had never thought about it that way. I have thought about it many times since that conversation, though.

I am thinking about it again now as I hear Louisa singing upstairs, her confident voice full of teenage hopes. It's possible that the moxie I so admire in my mom and my daughter did not skip a generation. It's possible that I possess the inner strength to stare cancer in the face and say, "Not now. Maybe not ever."

On behalf of the women who paved the way for me, and the generations to follow, I am ready to act. With a smile on my face and mischief in my hazel eyes, I will give cancer a sharp, debilitating, figurative kick in the nuts.

Sounds fair to me.

GRAND PRIZE WINNER

Katrina Smith, Burke, VA, she spent her childhood in Vermont woods and now lives in Burke VA with her husband, two children, three cats and a dog. When she's not writing she spends her time researching historical figures and making tea. Katrina holds a Bachelor of Arts degree in English with an emphasis on creative fiction from George Mason University and is currently pursuing a Masters of Fine Arts in Fiction from that same institution. She has been published in *Calliope: the Student Journal of Art and Literature*.

Judge Laurie Hertzel's comments on Covenant: This brief, poignant essay is written like poetry and filled with emotion—grief, fatalism, nostalgia, fear and hope. It rambles and frets, hopping from topic to topic, as our minds do when we are faced with an enormous problem. The rosebush, the rain, the playing children, the detritus of trash—all take on layers of meaning as the narrator's disease "makes holes like swiss cheese" inside of her and her center is weighed down "by pale stones." Such strong, lovely writing here, leaving the reader with much to think about.

FIRST PRIZE WINNER

Lynne Jonell, Plymouth, MN, is a children's writer who lives and works in Plymouth, Minnesota. She is married and the mother of two grown sons. She loves to sail, play the piano, and draw, and when she is feeling particularly virtuous she also manages to weed her garden. www.lynnejonell.com

Judge Laurie Hertzel's comments: The illness in this essay is a mother's dementia, and the narrator looks at it in a straightforward, tender way, laced with bitter humor. As the narrator comes to terms with her mother's illness, she also comes to terms with her mother—a classic mother-daughter relationship, complicated by illness. Nicely written, in a way that feels fresh and sad, not sentimental or pat.

FIRST HONORABLE MENTION

Susan Thurston, St. Paul, MN, is an author whose work is found in numerous publications including *Minnesota Monthly*, the Minneapolis *StarTribune*, anthologies including *Low Down and Coming On* (Red Dragonfly Press, 2011), and *Water's Edge* (Open to Interpretation, 2012), on-line in Garrison Keillor's "Writer's Almanac" (February 8, 2011), and at her blog www.susanthurstonwrites.com. Her *novel Sister of Grendel* will be published as an e-book in 2012, and she is at work on another novel with the working title, *The Comet and Clara*, along with several other writing projects. She lives with her family in St. Paul.

SECOND HONORABLE MENTION

Holly Harden.
At age nine, in the back seat of her grandmother's car on the way to a funeral, Holly Harden began to write, and she's been writing ever since. She grew up in several small Wisconsin towns, and majored in English and education at St. Olaf College in Northfield, Minnesota. In 2002, after teaching English and literature at the secondary level for nine years, she earned an MFA in writing from Hamline University. Her nonfiction work has appeared in publications such as *Utne* and *Fourth Genre*, and she is the editor for Garrison Keillor's *Life Among the Lutherans*. Holly lives in Forest Lake, Minnesota, where she writes for *A Prairie Home Companion*, teaches writing classes, and helps her three children get where they're going.

Katie Maxim, Duluth, MN. Biographic information was unavailable.

Sean James McGinty: Born and raised in San Bernardino CA. Educated at UCLA, Gonzaga University (English Lit & Philosophy), and Loyola-Marymount University's School of Film, and Weston School of Theology at Boston College (MTS). Moreover, Sean spent eleven years in the Jesuits and six living in Ireland. A five time marathon runner, Sean was recently diagnosed with Stage III Parkinson's disease.

Mary Rehwald lives in Ashland, Wisconsin, where she ran the Lifelong Learning Center at Northland College for many years. She brought many artists and writers to campus. She is very unofficially retired now. A night owl, she likes to write in the middle of the night. During the day, she carries little drawing books and watercolors around with her. She loves to fill them up. She served on the Ashland City Council for ten years, and has been a community organizer for over forty years. Social justice and sustainability drive her community work. She also sponsors house concerts in her home.

Jess Koski lives, for the time being, in a cabin outside of Two Harbors, Minnesota. He teaches English at Hibbing Community College.

Eugenie Doyle, Bristol, VT, author of two novels for young adults, *Stray Voltage* and *According to Kit* (Frontstreet/Boyds Mills Press) and many short stories, is a graduate of the VT College MFA in Writing program. She teaches frequently at the New England Young Writers conference at Breadloaf. She and her family operate The Last Resort, an organic berry, vegetable, and hay farm. In her spare time she practices and teaches yoga and paddles with Dragonheart Vermont.

Caren B. Stelson, Minneapolis, MN, continues to paddle down the "Great Snake River of Life" with her husband Kim, now recovered from colon cancer. With two grown children on their own, Caren focuses on her lifelong work as educator and author, writing mostly for children and young adults.

Jacqueline M. Rennwald, was born in St. Louis, MO, the second youngest of five children. She graduated from Gustavus Adolphus College intending to teach English but became a morning Disc Jockey for ten years. Jackie, her husband Charles, and son Henry met her husband, Charles, in 1997. They married in 2004, and their son Henry was born in 2004. Currently, Jackie and her family live in Two Harbors, Minnesota, where she is a stay-at-home mother, home schooling their son. A friend told her about the Kelly Culhane Writing Prize so she picked up her old habit of writing, starting work on a new project, and is once again writing fiction.

Teresa Boyle Falsani, born and raised in Portland, Maine, has lived in Duluth, Minnesota since 1973. A mother of two, she enjoyed second and third careers as creative director at Fochs and Associates Advertising and teaching English literature. Falsani is a winner of the 2011 Peace River Writers' Contest (Florida) and a two-time winner of Lake Superior Writers' Contests for her poetry and drama. Her writing has appeared in *Dust and Fire, Beloved on the Earth: 150 Poems of Grief and Gratitude, Migrations: Poetry and Prose for Life's Transitions*, and several other anthologies and journals.

Mary Lu Perham, Solon Springs, Wisconsin, is retired, but occasionally works as a musician playing the Celtic harp. Published work includes feature stories and news articles for magazines and newspapers. She currently writes fiction and creative non-fiction, which draw on her work in varied occupations, including security officer, welder, carpenter, carriage driver, university instructor and program coordinator.

Beverly Jovanovich, Andover, Minnesota, is interested in all of the arts. Writing, water-color, acrylic painting, and photography, but writing has been my strongest interest. I have done reporting for the *Anoka Union Newspaper*, the *Sun Newspaper* and the *Andover Express*. Interviewing people is the most interesting to me as one learns so much about different people that have unique things going on in their lives. I have a children's Christmas story that I am hoping to publish sometime in the future. I live in Andover, Minnesota and raised three sons.

Chuck Bransford, Stillwater, Minnesota: Thirty-one years of practice in general internal medicine in Stillwater, MN. Medical director Lakeview hospital Stillwater. Medical Director Lakeview hospice/palliative care. Two daughters, two grandsons, two dogs, and one very patient wife.

Connie Lounsbury, Monticello, Minnesota, is the author of five books, including her memoir *Thrift Store Shoes* released in January, 2012 by Inspiring Voices, a division of Guideposts. See www.connielounsbury.com for more information about her writing and inspirational speaking.

Shannon Esboldt, is a third grade teacher at South Washington County Schools, Royal Oaks Elementary, Cottage Grove, Minnesota.

Viola LaBounty, Solon Springs, Wisconsin, has been writing since her teen years, is a retired teacher's assistant, where she worked with children with autism. She is a married mother of two adult children, one teenage granddaughter and has a wonderful husband who is supportive of her writing. She is a member of Lake Superior Writer's Group, a Charter member of Wisconsin Writer's Association & St. Croix Writers, Solon Springs, Wisconsin.

Roxanne Wilmes lives in Duluth, Minnesota, with her husband, Mike, and mini Schnauzer, Fritz. Besides writing, she likes to spend time with her children and grandchildren, cook/bake, read, craft, and run. She is the VP of Marketing and Social Media for Fresh Air Lodging.

Mary Van Beusekom, BA, ELS, is a Minnesota-based writer, editor and marketing/communications professional with more than twenty years of experience working with consumer, physician and business audiences in print and online. After earning her BA in journalism and biology at the University of Minnesota, she worked as a newspaper reporter for five years until returning to college to complete her pre-med coursework. Since 2000, she has worked as a medical writer, editor, marketing/communications professional, and journalist. Originally from Loretto, Minn., she lives in Excelsior, Minn., with her husband, son and daughter.

James D. Rusin, M.D., MBA, Anoka, MN, has had a rather intense and exciting life as a practicing Family Physician, husband and father, polio survivor, mediator, and writer who was just was diagnosed with his third cancer. "These experiences and more have given me a unique and interesting perspective on life and very little time for self-pity. I am too busy living to worry about dying. Keep laughing, do not take yourself or anything else too seriously and you will get by and just maybe have as full a life as I have managed to have."

Elaine J. (Lohmeier) Fealy, Duluth, MN, is a counselor, foster parent, emergency chaplain, and an activist for children's rights. In 1981, she was presented with the Citizen of the Year Award for humanitarian services by the city of Columbia Heights, MN.

Kathy Tate, Duluth, MN, has been interested in social justice issues for decades, working in the psychotherapy field with children for over twenty-five years. She has been living with metastatic breast cancer since 2008, and soon after diagnosis left her professional field to travel and focus on her art and writing. She has most recently completed her first person obituary. *Kathy passed away on July 16, 2012.*

Jane Aas, Duluth, MN, is a self-taught musician that has recently discovered songwriting. A wife, mother of three, nurse, daughter, sister and friend, she finds inspiration in the lake, the moon, the environment, and time with others.

Marion Dane Bauer, is the author of more than eighty books for young people, ranging from novelty and picture books through early readers, both fiction and nonfiction, books on writing, and middle-grade and young-adult novels. She has won numerous awards, including several Minnesota Book Awards, a Jane Addams Peace Association Award for *Rain of Fire*, an American Library Association Newbery Honor Award for *On My Honor*, a number of state children's choice awards and the Kerlan Award from the University of Minnesota for the body of her work.

She is also the editor of and a contributor to the ground breaking collection of gay and lesbian short stories, *Am I Blue? Coming Out from the Silence*

Marion was one of the founding faculty and the first Faculty Chair for the Master of Fine Arts in Writing for Children and Young Adults program at Vermont College of Fine Arts. Her writing guide, the American Library Association Notable *What's Your Story? A Young Person's Guide to Writing Fiction*, is used by writers of all ages. Her books have been translated into more than a dozen different languages. She has six grandchildren and lives in St. Paul, Minnesota, with her partner and a cavalier King Charles spaniel, Dawn.

William McCarthy is from Stillwater, Minnesota. *The Arrival* appeared as *Breast Cancer Poem #1* in my chapbook, *Past Sins*, published by Trilobite Press at the University of North Texas as part of its Contemporary Poets Reading series. *Dark Companion* was published by *Main Channel Voices* literary magazine in Winona under the title, *Breast Cancer Poem #2*. The magazine also submitted it for a Pushcart Prize that year. It didn't win.

Cheryl Stratos lives in McLean, Virginia. She received a B.S. in Economics with a minor in Communications from George Mason University, and holds a Degree in Association publishing company *Innovative Association Solutions* in Alexandria, VA. Her focus is writing creative copy to sell programs and ad space for non-profits and develop creative fund raising programs. Her article *My Big C* has been published in *Viva Tysons* and she is currently working on launching the website named *Fighting Melanoma*. This will be a user-friendly survivor's manual for cancer patients and their families.

Atossa Shafaie lives in Sterling, VA. She received a B.A. in English literature from George Washington University. She is currently studying to get her MFA in creative writing at George Mason University. Born in Tehran, Iran and raised in America, her fiction aims to bridge the gap between the cultures of East and West. She has published the short stories *Mind the Gap* and *Woman to Woman*. Her short story *Growing Pains* will be published in the upcoming Fish Anthology and her flash fiction received honorable mention from Glimmer Train.

Donna Luby, Zimmerman, MN, Donna Luby's essay, "White Lies," was written as a tribute to her mother's memory. She resides with her husband, Dan, in rural Zimmerman, MN. She is a full time medical transcriber and is busy with children, grandchildren and their pets. She has rekindled her love of writing gaining support and encouragement from a writing group called *Word Weavers of Elk River*. Her writing is done in the quiet hours in late evenings and early mornings. She has contributed several pieces to Word Weavers' *Haunted House*, *Second Helpings*, and *Feast of Memories* thematic collections self-published by the Word Weavers'. She also has *Shadows* and *The Woodlanders* digitally published through Amazon on Kindle.

Lois K. Gibson, Minneapolis, Minnesota, studied at Ohio State University, is retired, and writes murder mysteries.

Carolyn Kluender's poetry, *Beekeepers Mosaic* has been published as part of a grant for the East Central Regional Library's 2012 poetry selections. Carolyn worked in the sign business, owned the Last Ditch Art Gallery in Stockholm, Wisconsin, worked nights as a bartender, all while raising her son. Recently, she is an artist mentor to Cambridge and North Branch area teens. She earned her BFA from College of Visual Arts in St Paul, Minnesota. Besides writing poetry, she paints watercolors, keeps bees, chickens, dogs and cats on a hobby farm north of Cambridge, Minnesota, and is a founding member of a women's writing group. Her mother died of breast cancer at age forty when she was fourteen, which made an impact that has been truly challenging to put into words. She promises her writing will only get better, she's thankful that people are patient enough to wade through her foray, and is thrilled to be included alongside writers with much more talent and more years of practice than she.

Nancy Roberts has been working as a registered nurse in the Operating Room for twenty-five years. She currently resides in Woodbury, Minnesota, with her husband Doug. They are parents to Rebeccah and Benjamin. Life is busy but finding the time to write is rewarding and therapeutic. Nancy is the self-published author of *Heaven Cent Prayers* and of numerous articles for church and hospital publications.

Heidi Schauer is a freelance writer and photographer who began storytelling before she could spell. At twelve, *What the American flag means to Me*, won first place in the Brainerd VFW Loyalty Day essay contest. By sixteen, she was a co-editor of her high school newspaper and attending Central Lakes College where she earned a degree emphasizing photography. She studied at Saint Cloud State University graduating in 2001 with a Bachelor of Science degree in Mass Communications. Passionate about people and places, she has published articles documenting her adventures with the Special Olympic World Winter Games in Anchorage, Alaska, Habitat for Humanity builds in Uganda and Kaua'i, and Minnesotans who have made a difference. Most recently, her travels have taken her to Ireland to explore her Cunningham family heritage. Schauer currently lives in Wyoming, Minnesota, with her husband and their two young children. She writes freelance articles and has started a blog, *A Heart's Thread*, (aheartsthread.wordpress.com) telling her tales.

Jean Steffenson, Onamia, Minnesota, has three sons and a daughter. Her daughter is still in high school. She has worked as a school speech/language pathologist (therapist/clinician) for over thirty years and is a strong advocate of prevention and early detection of skin cancer.

Rosanna Klepper: "Ever since my success in second grade with *The Dog,* I have been writing. My work has appeared in the *Chicago Sun-Times,* the *Chicago Tribune, Iowa City Magazine,* and the University of Iowa's award winning *Alumni Magazine.* I am a big fan of Ogden Nash and have written many witty Ditties. I have a blog, *The Accidental Nurse,* and I work as a freelance copyeditor and writer.

Judy Watson Tiesel, is no stranger to the dark companion of illness or grief, having grown up in a funeral home with parents whose mission was to be a comfort to grieving families. That background, along with her years as a minister's wife, catalyzed her interest in family dynamics. She taught Marriage & Family Therapy in three different graduate programs, and now continues in her MFT/Psychology private practice located in Edina, Minnesota, specializing in couples' issues and trauma. She was married for thirty-five years and has three inspiring children, all of whom provide richness for therapy, writing, and being present to life.

Christopher O. Moore writes essays and poetry in Belle Plaine, Minnesota. He retired from teaching high school English and directing theater in 2004, then worked for a time at a communications firm as an administrative assistant for several non-profits. Currently, his time is mostly devoted to his spouse LaVonne, their dogs Arlo and Guthrie, and keeping his drives in the fairway.

Kathleen Shega, Apple Valley, MN, was born in Zanesville, OH and grew up in Hopkins, MN. She graduated from St. Cloud State University. Following college, she joined Cargill in a Human Resources career. She and her family of three children spent four years in TX. She enjoys reading, crafts, biking, and walking.

Mara Hart, Duluth, MN, a native of New York, has lived in the Northland for over thirty years, where she writes memoir in prose and poetry, edits, and teaches. Among other places, her writing has been published in *Trail Guide, Lifeboat, Sing Heavenly Muse,* and the anthology, *When Last on the Mountain.* She co-edited *Beloved on the Earth,* edited *Lovecraft's New York Circle,* and is currently writing a memoir about her parents' first twelve years of marriage: *Lucy & George: The Bookshop Years.* She lives in Duluth with her cats, Roxie and Sophia.

Mary Martha Kobus, is originally from Lake Forest, IL, and is studying for an MFA in Fiction at George Mason University. She works for the U.S. Department of State. She is a graduate of Sarah Lawrence College and lives in Virginia with her husband and dog.

Patricia A. Gott teaches college composition and classes in British and Irish literature with an emphasis in gender studies at a public university in central Wisconsin. Patricia was born and raised in Superior, Wisconsin, and calls Lake Superior her spiritual home. She loves travel, local food, honest conversation and heartfelt music and is honored to be included in this volume of personal essays.

Lindsay Lee Johnson, Cambridge, MN, is an award-winning author of several books for children, including her latest picture book, *Ten Moonstruck Piglets.* For adults, she has published numerous essays, histories, and short fiction. Currently, she is pursuing her MFA in creative nonfiction at Hamline University in St. Paul, MN. She lives in the east central Minnesota countryside with her husband, two old chickens, two young cats, and a very bad dog.

Amy Padden grew up in Wisconsin but now lives in Minnesota with her husband and two little boys. She spends her days teaching and is working on her first novel.

Mary Amundsen, Rochester, MN, is a licensed psychologist, nurse, and grandmother. Among other successes, her poetry has appeared in *The Cancer Poetry Project,* which won the Minnesota Book Award for anthology in 2002.

Mary Jo McCarthy, resides in Northern Minnesota, with her husband, Tim, where they have enjoyed living at their lake home for the past thirty years. She counts herself blessed; having two married children and seven grandchildren all within easy visiting distance.

Mary Jo, a retired elementary teacher, enthusiastically writes short stories, inspirational pieces, biographies and tall tale adventures. Living on a peninsula, surrounded by three incredibly clear, sapphire-blue lakes, provides her the greatest incentive to give thanks always for His bountiful blessings.

Sharyl Saver, South St. Paul, was diagnosed with a recurrence of breast cancer that had spread to her lymph nodes and liver in May 2009. Sharyl shared her journey with poignant, honest, and, at times, humorous entries on her CaringBridge website. Hundreds followed her story. Sharyl lost her battle with cancer in July 2011. For information about the memoir based on her CaringBridge posts, visit www.fightlikeacowgirl.com. Her essay is reprinted with permission from *Fight Like a Cowgirl Press.*

Steve Linstrom, completed a career in state government and another as an executive in the corporate world. He's now focused on writing fiction while pursuing a graduate degree in English from Minnesota State University Mankato.

His work has appeared in the 2009 and 2010 *Arizona Literary Magazine* and the 2010 *Talking Stick Literary Journal.* Steve's novel *The Last Ram* was a quarterfinalist in the 2009 and 2010 Amazon.com Breakthrough Novel Contest and the short story *Lake Marshall* won the 2010 Brainerd Writers Contest. He and his wife Stephanie live in Marshall, Minnesota.

Micky McGilligan, Two Harbors, MN, has published poetry and essays for over thirty years in publications such as *Loonfeather, North Coast Review*, both Poetry Harbor regional anthologies, *Mother Earth News*, and translations from Spanish poetry in *Kalliope*, and have won awards from Lake Superior Writer's Series and Poetry Harbor.

Jeff Colla, Minneapolis, MN, was born and raised in Fond du Lac, Wisconsin and received his engineering degree from UW-Madison. He has spent the last thirty-five years in Minneapolis running his own business. Interests include; spending time at the lake, fishing, woodworking, and enjoying music.

Shari Albers has kept a journal since she was thirteen-years-old, often sketching within and around her words. Meeting and connecting at an arts workshop in 1980, Shari and Dorothy Sauber continued to write, draw, and share their journal pages until Dorothy died of lung cancer in 2008. Shari is a graphic artist and writer of local history, essays, and children's stories and lives with her family in South Minneapolis.

Brenda Hartman, was diagnosed with stage-IV ovarian cancer in 1988. She is a psychotherapist in private practice, specializing in oncology. Ms. Hartman presents programs locally and nationwide to cancer patients and their supporters. She is the author of, *Tell 'em Charlie Sent Ya*, and *The Golden Thread*. She lives in Falcon Heights, Minnesota with her family. Ms. Hartman can be reached through her web site: www.healingthroughlife.com.

Kelly Paradis, is the editor and writer of *Heartnotes Journal*, a quarterly publication educating consumers about hospice and palliative care. She has spent most of her life in Minnesota, except for a brief stint in Ottawa, Ontario running an Internet company with her husband during the 1990s dot-com boom. When she isn't writing or working on web projects, she spends her free time volunteering with therapy dog Chase in Twin Cities schools and libraries. She has been married to Mike for fifteen years and lives with two dogs and three cats.

Nathan R. Miller, is a writer and teacher in the southern Twin Cities area, where he lives with his inspiring wife and two young children. His memoir, *Teaching in Circles* (Kaplan 2008) explores his love/hate relationship with the first years of his high school English teaching career. He received his MFA from Hamline University, where he was fortunate enough to work with the editors of Water~Stone Review. He can be reached through his website at http://www.NathanRMiller.com

Deborah Gordon Cooper, Duluth, Minnesota, has been writing poetry for twenty years and has worked collaboratively with visual artists, musicians and dancers. She and her husband, Joel, who is a printmaker, have exhibited their collaborative images throughout the Midwest. Deborah has used poetry extensively in her work as a Hospice Chaplain. She co-edited the anthology, *Beloved on the Earth: 150 Poems of Grief & Gratitude*, (Holy Cow Press, 2009). She frequently teaches writing classes for those who are grieving the loss of a loved one. She conducts workshops on the interfacing of poetry and spirituality, and mentors inmates at the St. Louis County Jail. Deborah is the author of five collections of poems, most recently *Under the Influence of Lilacs* published by Clover Valley Press, May 2010.

Lynn J. McLean, St. Paul, MN, was born in Philadelphia, Pennsylvania, in 1945. She graduated from Millersville State University in Library Science and subsequently earned a Masters Degree in Curriculum and Instruction at Teachers College, Columbia University. Later, she received a Masters of Divinity from United Theological Seminary of the Twin Cities and was ordained in 1984. Lynn has been married to Gary for 44-years. They have six adult children, four of them Korean. They have six grandchildren.

Lynn has worked as a school librarian; home jewelry consultant; youth, Associate and Interim pastor; and Executive Director of a community-based health care service for the elderly.

Since Lynn's last surgery (5/2011), there has been no sign of cancer. She and Gary have returned to the global travel his job requires. Lynn is working on three books.

Katherine Morrow, Onamia, Minnesota, was born in Thief River Falls, Minnesota, attended Bemidji State University and received a Bachelor of Arts in 1977 and Master of Arts in English in 1981. She has lived in the Onamia area since then, working as an English teacher at Nay-Ah-Shing School on the Mille Lacs Reservation, Central Lakes College and Onamia High School. She and Jim Johnson were married in 1985 and have two daughters. Morrow has also worked as a Branch Librarian at Mille Lacs Lake Community Library in Isle, Minnesota since 2002.

Beret Griffith. After thirty years of writing for work as a facilitator, trainer and organization development consultant in large communities from coast to coast, my husband and I moved to the small town of Northfield, Minnesota in 2001. I joined a weekly writing group with a friend. The group has met weekly since 2003. It was also time to see if the art spirit had deserted me, after being in the background since the early 1970s. I went to the Women's Art Institute at the Minneapolis College of Art and Design in 2006. I've been writing, making art and taking snap shots ever since.

Nancy Maratta, Pittsboro, NC, is a lifetime devotee of the arts and humanities, Nan's thirty-year career in teaching and educational administration took her from the Northeast (NY, MA, and VT) to the Southwest (Arizona) and finally, the southwest delta of Bush Alaska. Her most coveted award was *Outstanding Teacher of the Year* at Pima County Community College in 1987, as it was a student generated, college-wide award. Widely read in continental philosophy and twentieth century literature, her favorite genre is poetry. Cross-country skiing, dragon boating, hiking and healthy cooking occupy Nan's free time. She and her husband, Gene, with dogs Maggie and Murphy in tow, divide their time between the blue skies of North Carolina and the mountains and lakes of New York and Vermont.

Carol Germ, Brooklyn Park, Minnesota, enjoys observing and putting into words what has happened not only in her life but also with the people she has known, helped, and befriended throughout her life and career. "I am at present retired from a forty-year career as a registered nurse. My years of being present in this life have been full of good stories, funny stories and some sad stories. They have all stimulated growth and maybe even some wisdom."

Adele L. Bergstrom, Minneapolis, MN, is a designer and writer at A. Light Communications in Minneapolis. As a grant recipient of the 2006 *SAPPI Ideas that Matter Campaign*, Adele designed and edited the book *Who Asked Me: A Journal of Discovery Sharing By and For Siblings of People with Developmental Disabilities*. She and her husband have three children, the youngest of whom has Down syndrome. In 2003, the writer underwent treatment for breast cancer—an experience that left her committed to the philosophy of living one day at a time. Adele continues to write and advocate on issues relevant to breast cancer as well as those impacting the disability community.

Teresa Kleinschmidt, Spring Lake Park, MN, has lived with Type I Diabetes for thirty years. She works as a family therapist with kids and adolescents living with chronic illness in the Minneapolis area. She has one twelve-year-old daughter who can't wait to jump in the lake next New Year's Day!

Kristine Zimmer Orkin, Whitefish Bay, WI, The eldest of six siblings, Kris was born into a large and loving extended family of German and Irish descent, and has lived her entire life in Wisconsin. She left the security of her small Menasha hometown in 1976 and ventured into an urban metropolis to attend the University of Wisconsin-Milwaukee, the only in-state school then offering a degree in Deaf Education. Kris is a licensed special education teacher and a nationally certified sign language interpreter. She specializes in educational, religious, and theatrical interpreting. Kris still resides in Milwaukee, where she met and married Philip Orkin, the man with the "Betty Grable legs". Together for twenty-six years, they added three sons to their family tree—Joseph, Jacob, and Jonathan. Little Jacob was already waiting at Heaven's door, excited to welcome his daddy Home in June of 1997. We are indeed blessed.
"To everything there is a season, and a time to every purpose . . ." (Ecclesiastes 3:1)

Jeanne Marie Riese, is a self-employed financial analyst living on Upper Eau Claire Lake in the Town of Barnes, WI. Jeanne writes, creates tiles, pottery, sculpture, and silk paintings, with a focus on healing, nature, beauty and love. Jeanne can be reached at jeannemarie@jeannemariedesigns.com, or at her studio in Barnes. Her overall attitude toward art and life is: Live Big, Love Big.

Linda Kirchmaier, Duluth, MN, is a seasoned soul and a novice poet with words and reflections waiting within to show up on paper. She is a life-long learner and has always lived in Minnesota. Her love of Lake Superior and its surrounding nature have kept her in Duluth for over forty years. Her retirement career is that of being a Life Coach. This is her first publication. She is a fifteen-month survivor of salivary gland cancer.

Keith Johnson, is a Media Technology Director at Bloomington Kennedy High School. Keith and his wife Ann live in New Prague, Minnesota, and have four children: Geoff, Jenna, Maria, and Anna. In addition to teaching and coaching, he is an avid musician and plays acoustic Americana music on 6-string and 12-string guitars, on various sizes of mandolins, and blows and sucks on harmonica, sometimes creating some semblance of music. He is the "prairie dog" half of the musical duo *Celtic Cat & Prairie Dog*, appropriately so, since he hails from the verdant western prairie of Benson, Minnesota.

Rachel Nelson, Two Harbors, Minnesota, is a storyteller, songwriter, and musician whose passion is live performance. She sparks her stories with physical acting techniques, and often acts as her own "theater musician."

Margaret Manderfeld, Duluth, Minnesota, is involved in many ways to express herself through the arts. Seeking truth and beauty, she is inspired by nature and is compelled to "vent" her observations. Her writing often aims for a humorous perspective, wanting the reader to find a poignant meaning within the whimsy.

Andrea Oberg-McArdle, started out writing short stories and poetry for adults, but the birth of her first son renewed her passion for children's literature. Three boys later she is still writing poetry, but also finds joy in writing and illustrating for a younger audience. Picture books may be her favorite form, but poetry will forever be her first love.

Andrea holds a Bachelor's Degree in Art with an emphasis in Graphic Design from the University of Wisconsin-Madison. She was the recipient of the 2009 Shabo Award for Children's Picture Book Writers from The Loft Literary Center and continues to write in her spare time. While most of her day is spent raising three exuberant little boys, she also runs a home-based Graphic and Web Design Studio, Grebo Design. She currently lives in Forest Lake, Minnesota, with her wonderful husband and children.

Lizzy Carney, is a writer, educator, reader, and traveler. She has the vision that learning is a lifelong expedition and embraces detours. Lizzy believes in allowing ourselves the avenues and winding roads to discover possibilities. She meets with an array of inspired individuals to explore writing, creativity and literature. As an adjunct professor at Antioch University, her teaching focus is with adults who are studying for their special education endorsements or completing their Master's degrees. Additionally, Lizzy offers courses for elementary school teachers through the Heritage Institute. Her classes assist teachers to use children's picture books to enhance instruction in writing and the content areas. She enjoys writing in a variety of genres: stories for children's picture books, poetry, cookbooks and has notebooks of ideas for inspiration for her next project. Lizzy is a member of the Society of Children's Book Writers and Illustrators. She holds a Master's degree from Antioch University—Seattle and a Bachelors from Gonzaga University.

Linda L. Klein, Stillwater, Minnesota, has facilitated a weekly support group for women with recurrent cancer for the past 14-years at St. John's Hospital in Maplewood, MN, a part of the HealthEast Care System. Prior to starting the support group, she authored two books published by John Wiley of New York: *I Can Cope: Staying Healthy with Cancer* and *The Support*

Group Sourcebook. For the past twelve years, she has also been the conference coordinator for a cancer survivorship conference hosted by HealthEast, *The Many Faces of Hope.* After staying home to raise three children, she lives with her husband Bill in an "empty nest" on a hobby farm north of Stillwater, Minnesota.

B. J. Johnson, is a professional communicator who resides in Minneapolis, Minnesota. His background includes work in journalism and corporate communications. His work has appeared in the *Star Tribune* newspaper and various magazines. He is an avid traveler. In his spare time, he is a wild mushroom hunter.

Mary Sweere, was born, raised, and graduated from high school in Glenwood, Minnesota. In 1964, she graduated from St. Mary's School of Nursing and became a Registered Nurse. Mary and her husband Joe reside in Owatonna, Minnesota and have six grown children. When she learned of the melanoma in her left eye, she was inspired to write and publish her first book, *Forgive Me Father.* She has since completed writing her fourth book.

Paul H. Waytz, M.D., is a native of Chicago and attended Washington University in St. Louis as an undergraduate and University of Illinois for medical school. He moved to Minneapolis in 1973 for his residency and subsequent fellowship in Rheumatology. Dr. Waytz has been in private practice for over thirty years and enjoys ranting about the changes in medicine he has observed. His outside interests include exercise, gardening, reading, and cheering for the usually hapless Chicago sports teams much to the annoyance of his wife and three sons. He aspires to be a very good writer.

Sandra Frederiksen Weicht: Elementary school teachers instilled in me the love of writing. My high school English teacher encouraged it. When my high school sweetheart returned from Vietnam, we married and settled in his hometown of Elk River, Minnesota where we grew our family and a construction company. We have four kids, two by birth and two by marriage; five of the best looking and smartest grand kids in the world, and wonderful family and friends. Word Weavers, my writers' group, has helped me finish projects that would have never become reality. The help, support, editing, and friendship enable the creative process to bloom.

My life has been touched by cancer in many ways. My mom had colon cancer, lung cancer and died of acute myelogenous leukemia, one of my husbands' brothers and two brothers-in-law died of cancer, my husband has chronic lymphocytic leukemia and esophageal cancer, and I had a double mastectomy for breast cancer. Too many of our family and friends have or had cancer.

The love of a Christian family and friends along with our community, has sustained me through hard times. God's angels' wings have surrounded and upheld us.

Life is wonderful. God is good.

Rachel D. Nemitz. Born at Box, Oklahoma, Rachel's was one of the many "Okie" families who moved to California during the 1930s and early 40s in search of a better life. She met and married, Richard, a Marine from Minnesota. They raised seven children on a hobby farm near Cologne, MN. A retired executive secretary, Rachel now resides in Buffalo, Minnesota, where she is a member of the Senior Writing group and serves on the Buffalo Library Board.

Paula Nelson-Guenther, has lived in Duluth, Minnesota since 1969, retiring in 2001 after having taught kindergarten through college music for forty-two years in Missouri, Illinois and Minnesota, but always remaining active in the music community.

Amy Lindgren is a business writer and career counselor by trade. She writes a nationally syndicated job search column *Working Strategies* and operates Prototype Career Service in St. Paul, Minnesota. She and her husband Bruce live in St. Paul and enjoy rehabbing old homes.

Bonnie Gintis, Winooski, VT, is living with metastatic breast cancer as an Osteopathic Physician, a Mindfulness Based Stress Reduction (MBSR) teacher, and an Authorized Continuum Movement teacher. She combines these approaches to explore applications in many aspects of life: self-care, health care, education, creativity, communication, and community. She is the author of *Engaging The Movement Of Life*.

Kirsten Young, Elk River, MN, grew up on a family farm in Ottertail County, Minnesota. After earning a B.S. in Vocal Music Education from Moorhead State University (MN), she moved to Washington State with her husband and four-year-old son. She earned an M.P.A. at Pacific Lutheran University. After a long career as a human services and public health professional in state and county government in Washington, North Dakota, Wisconsin and Minnesota, she retired to focus on getting well. She now shares a home in Elk River, Minnesota, with her daughter and nine year old grandson, Brock. Kirsten continues to work on her memoir and genealogy activities as a legacy for Brock.

Joy Fisher lives with her husband, four daughters and her maltipoo, Maggie. She enjoys living in Minnesota where she camps all summer and spends her winters reading mysteries.

Lisa McKhann, lives and writes in Duluth, Minnesota, where she has produced many mixed-art events. After treatment for ovarian cancer, she began a project for online reflective writing and selective reading for survivors. It's called JOMMA: Journal of My Medical Associations, and can be viewed at www.projectlulu.com.

Kate Severson, Lacey, WA, is a thirty year veteran of the Washington State Transportation Department, where she spins engineering content into creative technical manuals. After her bout with cancer in 2010, she pledged to spend her energy and resources into creative fiction, nonfiction, poetry and flash fiction. She is now rewarded by my "gift of cancer" to discover and implement her writing passion.

She has three kids, ranging from adult to adolescent. "I live for my family, writing group, book club and politics, as well as my pub mates at the Fish Brewing. Words are precious."

Jeske Noordergraaf: My parents came to the United States from the Netherlands, when I was two-years-old. I was one of four children and I grew up with an interest in science which I got from my father, who is a biophysicist. From my mother, a social worker, I learned about helping others and that not everyone is equally fortunate. We spent several Christmases as a family serving dinner at homeless shelters. I have loved animals from an early age and my dream was to be a veterinarian. I attended the University of Pennsylvania both for my undergraduate degree and my veterinary degree. After graduation, I worked in veterinary practices both in Pennsylvania and Minnesota before starting my own practice here in 1995, Sunrise Equine Veterinary Services. I married my husband, Jim who is a Minnesota native in 1994 and my son Clay was born in 1996. I was diagnosed with breast cancer in Dec 2005. I was able to keep my business going during my ten-month treatment and from this I learned a great deal about health care and the costs.

Kris Brenna Lyons, grew up in Proctor, Minnesota, and has always proven the statement, "Diamonds are a girl's best friend, softball diamonds that is!" Whether playing or umpiring, she has always reached for excellence in the great game of softball. As a kid playing in the neighborhood with the boys or the summer spent in her grandma's back yard, she could be heard giving suggestions to her teammates or instructions on calls or rules, sometimes to the point where she was sent to her bedroom to think about what she had screamed throughout the neighborhood. She could be heard more than once expressing her opinion, "But I'm trying to help. It's a rule, but they just don't play by the rules!" Cancer is like that, not playing by any rules, yet it can be overcome. She has been cancer free for over five years and is enjoying retirement after teaching English for thirty-five years, mostly in Moose Lake, Minnesota. "I am so busy, how did I ever work?"

Carol A. Schreier, is a mostly retired clinical social worker who lives, gardens, writes, and does yoga and some teaching in Minneapolis, Minnesota. She continues to remain clear of a re-occurrence of the ovarian cancer she experienced in 1999.

Mary Alice Harrold is an enrolled member of the White Earth Band of Ojibwe, White Earth, Minnesota. She is active in the native communities of the Twin Cities of Minneapolis and St. Paul and the White Earth reservation. She works in social services for a non-profit located in Minneapolis assisting clients with mental and chemical health issues obtain stability. Mary is a graduate of the University of Minnesota with a Journalism and Human Services background. She resumed her creative writing career in 2010 and has been involved in classes at the Loft Literary Center, the Loft sponsored TGIFrybread native writing group, as well as a weekly writing group working with Loft educator Roxanne Sadovsky.

Carol Larson was a teacher at St. Louis Park, Minnesota, high school and has written three books, *When the Trip Changes, Positive Options for Colorectal Cancer,* and *Lifelines.* Carol lives in Minnetonka, Minnesota, with her husband, Dave. They have six grandchildren.

Brenda Martin-Granstra, Heron Lake, Minnesota. Biographic information was unavailable.

Dorothy Sauber was well known in the 1980s for her vivid pictorial hooked rugs that illustrated ordinary family life, her rural Minnesota roots, and her community, as well as progressive politics and women's issues. As a college professor, Dorothy taught women's studies, African studies, world literature, and creative writing. She was a voracious reader and disciplined writer. When diagnosed with stage IV non-small cell lung cancer, Dorothy responded by creating a series of 16 essays that explored the many facets of living with a terminal disease. After her death, her sons and friends published *Cancer Essays: Not the Book I Was Planning to Write,* available at www.dorothysauber.com. She died of lung cancer in 2008 and the works herein were used with permission.

Joy Riggs, is a freelance journalist and an award-winning columnist for *Minnesota Parent* magazine. Her work has appeared in numerous publications including the *Star Tribune, Minnesota Monthly,* and *AAA Living.* She's also the copy editor for the *Voice,* the Carleton College alumni magazine. She lives in Northfield, Minn., with her husband, Steve, and their three children.